T0226609

Vascular Medicine

Editors

GENO J. MERLI
RAGHU KOLLURI

MEDICAL CLINICS
OF NORTH AMERICA

www.medical.theclinics.com

Consulting Editor
JACK ENDE

September 2023 • Volume 107 • Number 5

ELSEVIER

1600 John F. Kennedy Boulevard • Suite 1800 • Philadelphia, Pennsylvania, 19103-2899

http://www.theclinics.com

MEDICAL CLINICS OF NORTH AMERICA Volume 107, Number 5
September 2023 ISSN 0025-7125, ISBN-13: 978-0-443-12977-3

Editor: Taylor Hayes
Developmental Editor: Malvika Shah

Medical Clinics of North America (ISSN 0025-7125) is published bimonthly by Elsevier Inc., 360 Park Avenue South, New York, NY 10010-1710. Months of publication are January, March, May, July, September, and November. Business and editorial offices: 1600 John F. Kennedy Boulevard, Suite 1800, Philadelphia, PA 19103-2899. Periodicals postage paid at New York, NY, and additional mailing offices. Subscription prices are USD $332.00 per year (US individuals), $786.00 per year (US institutions), $100.00 per year (US Students), $416.00 per year (Canadian individuals), $1023.00 per year (Canadian institutions), $200.00 per year for (foreign students), $100.00 per year for (Canadian students), $461.00 per year (foreign individuals), and $1023.00 per year (foreign institutions). To receive student/resident rate, orders must be accompanied by name of affiliated institution, date of term, and the signature of program/residency coordinator on institution letterhead. Orders will be billed at individual rate until proof of status is received. Foreign air speed delivery is included in all Clinics' subscription prices. All prices are subject to change without notice. **POSTMASTER:** Send address changes to *Medical Clinics of North America*, Elsevier Health Sciences Division, Subscription Customer Service, 3251 Riverport Lane, Maryland Heights, MO 63043. **Customer Service: Telephone: 1-800-654-2452** (U.S. and Canada); **1-314-447-8871** (outside U.S. and Canada). **Fax: 314-447-8029. E-mail: journalscustomerserviceusa@ elsevier.com** (for print support); **journalsonlinesupport-usa@elsevier.com** (for online support).

Reprints. For copies of 100 or more of articles in this publication, please contact the Commercial Reprints Department, Elsevier Inc., 360 Park Avenue South, New York, NY 10010-1710. Tel.: 212-633-3874; Fax: 212-633-3820; E-mail: reprints@elsevier.com.

Medical Clinics of North America is also published in Spanish by McGraw-Hill Interamericana Editores S. A., P.O. Box 5-237, 06500 Mexico, D.F., Mexico.

Medical Clinics of North America is covered in *MEDLINE/PubMed (Index Medicus), Current Contents, ASCA, Excerpta Medica, Science Citation Index,* and *ISI/BIOMED.*

PROGRAM OBJECTIVE
The goal of the *Medical Clinics of North America* is to keep practicing physicians up to date with current clinical practice by providing timely articles reviewing the state of the art in patient care.

TARGET AUDIENCE
All practicing physicians and other healthcare professionals.

LEARNING OBJECTIVES
Upon completion of this activity, participants will be able to:
1. Review the process of atherosclerosis formation and factors contributing to the disease process.
2. Explain why peripheral artery disease remains an under-recognized and under-treated entity.
3. Discuss the prevalence and incidence of venous thromboembolism and predisposing risk factors of varicose veins.

ACCREDITATION
The Elsevier Office of Continuing Medical Education (EOCME) is accredited by the Accreditation Council for Continuing Medical Education (ACCME) to provide continuing medical education for physicians.

The EOCME designates this journal-based CME activity for a maximum of 11 *AMA PRA Category 1 Credit*(s)™. Physicians should claim only the credit commensurate with the extent of their participation in the activity.

All other healthcare professionals requesting continuing education credit for this enduring material will be issued a certificate of participation.

DISCLOSURE OF CONFLICTS OF INTEREST
The EOCME assesses conflict of interest with its instructors, faculty, planners, and other individuals who are in a position to control the content of CME activities. All relevant conflicts of interest that are identified are thoroughly vetted by EOCME for fair balance, scientific objectivity, and patient care recommendations. EOCME is committed to providing its learners with CME activities that promote improvements or quality in healthcare and not a specific proprietary business or a commercial interest.

The planning committee, staff, authors, and editors listed below have identified no financial relationships or relationships to products or devices they or their spouse/life partner have with commercial interest related to the content of this CME activity:
Aaron W. Aday, MD, MSc; James B. Alexander, MD, FACS, DFSVS; Matthew Bierowski, MD; G. Jay Bishop, MD; Eri Fukaya, MD, PhD; Michelle Littlejohn; Anthony Joseph Macchiavelli, MD, SFHM, FACP; Amry Majeed, MD; Geno J. Merli, MD, MACP, FSVM, FHM; Kunal Mishra, DO; Alireza Mofid, MD; Amanda M. Morrison, MD; Hunter Mwansa, MBBS; Craig Nielsen, MD; Dina Orapallo, MSN, CRNP, AGACNP-BC; Merlin Packiam; Randy Ramcharitar, MD; Ammar A. Saati, MD; Viviane Seki Sassaki, MD, RPVI, RVT, RDMS; Alexander E. Sullivan, MD; Heather Yenser, MSN, CRNP, AGACNP-BC; Mohamed Zghouzi, MD

The planning committee, staff, authors, and editors listed below have identified financial relationships or relationships to products or devices they or their spouse/life partner have with commercial interest related to the content of this CME activity:
Geoffrey D. Barnes, MD, MSc: Consultant: Abbott, Bayer, Boston Scientific, Bristo-Myers Squibb, Janssen Pharmaceuticals, Pfizer.

Taki Galanis, MD: Consultant: Janssen Pharmaceuticals.

Daniella Kadian-Dodov, MD: Speaker: Abbott, Boston Scientific, MedScape, McGraw Hill; Researcher: Philips.

Raghu Kolluri, MD: Consultant: Abbott, Auxetics, Boston Scientific, Diachii Sankyo, Koya Medical, Medtronic, NAMSA, Penumbra, Philips, PERC, Surmodics, USA Therm, VB Devices.

Aditya Sharma, MD: Researcher: Boston Scientific, Vascular Medcure; Speaker: Boston Scientific.

UNAPPROVED/OFF-LABEL USE DISCLOSURE
The EOCME requires CME faculty to disclose to the participants;
1. When products or procedures being discussed are off-label, unlabelled, experimental, and/or investigational (not US Food and Drug Administration [FDA] approved); and
2. Any limitations on the information presented, such as data that are preliminary or that represent ongoing research, interim analyses, and/or unsupported opinions. Faculty may discuss information about

pharmaceutical agents that is outside of FDA-approved labelling. This information is intended solely for CME and is not intended to promote off-label use of these medications. If you have any questions, contact the medical affairs department of the manufacturer for the most recent prescribing information.

TO ENROLL

To enroll in the *Medical Clinics of North America* Continuing Medical Education program, call customer service at 1-800-654-2452 or sign up online at http://www.theclinics.com/home/cme. The CME program is available to subscribers for an additional annual fee of USD 282.00.

METHOD OF PARTICIPATION

In order to claim credit, participants must complete the following;
1. Complete enrolment as indicated above.
2. Read the activity.
3. Complete the CME Test and Evaluation. Participants must achieve a score of 70% on the test. All CME Tests and Evaluations must be completed online.

CME INQUIRIES/SPECIAL NEEDS

For all CME inquiries or special needs, please contact elsevierCME@elsevier.com.

MEDICAL CLINICS OF NORTH AMERICA

Contributors

CONSULTING EDITOR

JACK ENDE, MD, MACP
The Schaeffer Professor of Medicine, Perelman School of Medicine, University of Pennsylvania, Philadelphia, Pennsylvania

EDITORS

GENO J. MERLI, MD, MACP, FSVM, FHM
Professor of Medicine and Surgery, Co-Director, Jefferson Vascular Center, Director, Division of Vascular Medicine, Sidney Kimmel Medical College, Thomas Jefferson University Hospitals, Philadelphia, Pennsylvania

RAGHU KOLLURI, MD, MS, RVT
System Medical Director, Vascular Medicine and Vascular Laboratories, OhioHealth Heart and Vascular, Clinical Professor of Medicine, Ohio University HCOM, Columbus, Ohio

AUTHORS

AARON W. ADAY, MD, MSc
Assistant Professor of Medicine, Division of Cardiovascular Medicine, Department of Medicine, Vanderbilt Translational and Clinical Cardiovascular Research Center, Vanderbilt University Medical Center, Nashville, Tennessee

JAMES B. ALEXANDER, MD, FACS, DFSVS
Professor of Surgery, Division Vascular Medicine, Jefferson Vascular Center, Sidney Kimmel Medical College, Thomas Jefferson University, Philadelphia, Pennsylvania

GEOFFREY D. BARNES, MD, MSC
Frankel Cardiovascular Center, University of Michigan, Ann Arbor, Michigan

MATTHEW BIEROWSKI, MD
Resident, Internal Medicine, Thomas Jefferson University Hospital, Philadelphia, Pennsylvania

GERALD JAY BISHOP, MD
Associate Section Head, Section of Vascular Medicine, Cleveland Clinic, Cleveland, Ohio

ERI FUKAYA, MD, PhD
Clinical Associate Professor, Division of Vascular Surgery, Stanford University School of Medicine, Stanford, California

TAKI GALANIS, MD
Associate Professor of Medicine and Surgery, Division Vascular Medicine, Jefferson Vascular Center, Sidney Kimmel Medical College, Philadelphia, Pennsylvania

ANTHONY JOSEPH MACCHIAVELLI, MD, SFHM, FACP, RPVI
Clinical Assistant Professor of Vascular Medicine, Division Vascular Medicine, Jefferson Vascular Center, Sidney Kimmel Medical College, Philadelphia, Pennsylvania

DANIELLA KADIAN-DODOV, MD, FACC, FAHA, FSVM, RPVI
Assistant Professor of Medicine, Zena and Michael A. Wiener Cardiovascular Institute, Icahn School of Medicine at Mount Sinai, New York, New York

AMRY MAJEED, MD
Resident, Internal Medicine, Thomas Jefferson University Hospital, Philadelphia, Pennsylvania

GENO J. MERLI, MD, MACP, FSVM, FHM
Professor of Medicine and Surgery, Co-Director, Jefferson Vascular Center, Director, Division of Vascular Medicine, Sidney Kimmel Medical College, Thomas Jefferson University Hospitals, Philadelphia, Pennsylvania

KUNAL MISHRA, DO
Division of Cardiovascular Medicine, University of Virginia, Charlottesville, Virginia

ALIREZA MOFID, MD
Fellow, Vascular Surgery, Thomas Jefferson University Hospital, Philadelphia, Pennsylvania

AMANDA M. MORRISON, MD
Division of Cardiovascular Medicine, Department of Medicine, Vanderbilt University Medical Center, Nashville, Tennessee

HUNTER MWANSA, MBBS
Frankel Cardiovascular Center, University of Michigan, Ann Arbor, Michigan

CRAIG NIELSEN, MD
Vice Chair, Internal Medicine and Geriatrics, Department of Internal Medicine, Cleveland Clinic, Cleveland, Ohio

DINA ORAPALLO, MSN, CRNP, AGACNP-BC
Division of Vascular Medicine, Department of Surgery, Sidney Kimmel Medical College, Thomas Jefferson University Hospitals, Philadelphia, Pennsylvania

RANDY K. RAMCHARITAR, MD
Division of Cardiovascular Medicine, University of Virginia, Charlottesville, Virginia

AMMAR A. SAATI, MD
Staff Physician, Section of Vascular Medicine, Cleveland Clinic, Cleveland, Ohio

VIVIANE SEKI SASSAKI, MD, RPVI, RVT, RDMS
Senior Vascular Sonographer, Stanford Heart and Vascular Clinic - Vascular Laboratory, Stanford, California

ADITYA M. SHARMA, MD
Division of Cardiovascular Medicine, University of Virginia, Charlottesville, Virginia

ALEXANDER E. SULLIVAN, MD
Division of Cardiovascular Medicine, Department of Medicine, Vanderbilt University Medical Center, Nashville, Tennessee

HEATHER YENSER, MSN, CRNP, AGACNP-BC
Division of Vascular Medicine, Department of Surgery, Sidney Kimmel Medical College,
Thomas Jefferson University Hospitals, Philadelphia, Pennsylvania

MOHAMED ZGHOUZI, MD
Frankel Cardiovascular Center, University of Michigan, Ann Arbor, Michigan

Contents

Atherosclerotic disease, including stroke and myocardial infarction, is the leading cause of morbidity and mortality worldwide. Atherosclerotic plaque formation occurs in the setting of excess oxidative and hemodynamic stress and is perpetuated by smoking, poor diet, dyslipidemia, hypertension, and diabetes. Plaque may rupture, resulting in acute thrombotic events. Smoking cessation, lifestyle modification, risk factor optimization, and antithrombotic therapies are the mainstays of atherosclerotic disease management and are the cornerstones to reduce morbidity and mortality in this high-risk patient population. Novel therapeutics are in development and will add to the growing armamentarium available to physicians who manage atherosclerotic disease.

Peripheral artery disease (PAD) affects approximately 230 million people worldwide and is associated with an increased risk of major adverse cardiovascular and limb events. Even though this condition is considered a cardiovascular equivalent, it remains an underrecognized and undertreated entity. Antiplatelet and statin therapy, along with smoking cessation, are the foundations of therapy to reduce adverse events but are challenging to fully implement in this patient population. Race and socioeconomic status also have profound impacts on PAD outcomes.

Peripheral artery disease (PAD) affects approximately 230 million people worldwide and is associated with an increased risk of major adverse cardiovascular and limb events. Even though this condition is considered a cardiovascular equivalent, it remains an under-recognized and under-treated entity. Anti-platelet and statin therapy, along with smoking cessation, are the foundations of therapy to reduce adverse events but are challenging to fully implement in this patient population. Race and socioeconomic status also have profound impacts on PAD outcomes. Exercise therapy is the gold standard treatment of claudication while revascularization procedures are often reserved for patients with limb-threatening ischemia.

Raynaud's phenomenon is an exaggerated response to cold stimuli that may be primary or secondary. The diagnosis relies on patient history and physical examination to distinguish RP from other vasomotor dysfunction (e.g. acrocyanosis, pernio, small fiber neuropathy with vasomotor symptoms, and complex regional pain syndrome). Achenbach syndrome, or spontaneous venous hemorrhage, may also be mistaken for RP but is a self-limiting phenomenon. Laboratory evaluation and vascular diagnostic testing may identify SRP causes. Regardless of etiology, treatment includes warming with trigger avoidance, and consideration of vasodilators (eg. calcium channel, alpha-1 blockers). SRP with digital ulceration may require PDE5i, endothelin-1 receptor blockers, and prostanoids. Refractory cases may require pneumatic arterial pumps, botulinum toxin administration, or surgical sympathectomy.

Vasculitis is a diverse group of disorders involving inflammation of the blood vessels. Approaching the diagnosis of vasculitis can be challenging, given the differing clinical presentation and organ manifestations. Often vasculitis is a diagnosis that is considered too late, given the heterogeneous presentation and various mimics. This article aims to provide physicians with a diagnostic approach to vasculitis.

Venous thromboembolism (VTE) is a common vascular disorder encompassing deep vein thrombosis (DVT) and pulmonary embolism (PE). There is no data on global estimates of VTE prevalence and incidence. Most patients with unprovoked VTE require secondary thromboprophylaxis upon the completion of the primary treatment phase if they have no high bleeding risk. Risk prediction models can help identify patients at low VTE recurrence risk who may discontinue anticoagulation upon the completion of the primary treatment phase.

The Centers for Disease Control and Prevention estimates that approximately 900,000 patients are diagnosed with venous thromboembolism (VTE) annually in the United States leading to approximately 548,000 hospitalizations and 100,000 deaths. Approximately 274 people die daily in the United States from VTE. The numbers are staggering with 1 person dying every 5 minutes! There are more deaths annually in the United States from VTE than breast cancer (41,000), AIDS (16,000), and motor vehicle accidents (32,000) combined! VTE is recognized as a leading cause of preventable hospital deaths and a leading cause of maternal deaths.

Foreword

Why Not Vascular Medicine?

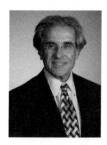

Jack Ende, MD, MACP
Consulting Editor

Subspecialties of internal medicine, such as cardiology, gastroenterology, endocrinology, and infectious diseases, tend to emerge when the corpus of information within a particular field reaches a critical mass such that professionals, either wittingly or maybe before they even appreciate it, find themselves thoroughly engaged. Moreover, the emergence of new theoretic and applied knowledge, particularly within therapeutics, demands that full engagement.[1] These nascent subspecialists then begin to publish in that field; they form societies and perhaps establish journals, and they begin to offer advanced training, such as fellowships; Eventually, they appeal to recognized specialty boards, such as the American Board of Internal Medicine or the American Board of Surgery, for recognition as a subspecialty complete with certification and accreditation of training programs.

Take for example infectious diseases, the history of which is insightfully presented by one of its most prominent leaders, the late Edward H. Kass, MD.[2] Kass argues that it was only after the advent of specific chemotherapeutic treatments and discoveries in microbiology and immunology that infectious diseases could become a subspecialty composed of physicians particularly knowledgeable in the increasing number of therapeutic and preventive measures for treating such diseases. More specifically, infectious diseases became a subspecialty when our understanding of its clinical problems evolved to the level of complexity demanding of academic physicians' full engagement, and when the therapies became effective enough that they came to be considered mainstream for patient care.

Are we at that stage in vascular medicine? The answer, I believe, is found in this issue of *Medical Clinics of North America*, "Vascular Medicine for Internists, Family Practitioners, and Advanced Practice Providers." Reflecting the specialized knowledge of its Guest Editors, Geno J. Merli and Raghu Kolluri, and the selected, expert authors, it includes articles on pathogenesis, diagnosis, clinical presentations, and approaches to management of an array of disorders from peripheral artery disease to

Med Clin N Am 107 (2023) xv–xvi
https://doi.org/10.1016/j.mcna.2023.06.006
0025-7125/23/© 2023 Published by Elsevier Inc.

venous thromboembolism, from ulcers to edema. These are the problems our patients bring to us in our practices, and these are the problems for which we are often dependent on our colleagues who have developed special knowledge and wisdom in these disorders, and who have devoted themselves to this fast-emerging field. Sounds like a subspecialty to me.

I hope this issue is useful to those of us in practice who so often find ourselves turning to our subspecialty colleagues for up-to-date information that we may apply.

Jack Ende, MD, MACP
Perelman School of Medicine of the
University of Pennsylvania
Philadelphia, PA, USA

E-mail address:
jack.ende@pennmedicine.upenn.edu

REFERENCES

1. Beeson PB. The natural history of medical subspecialties. Ann Int Med 1980;93: 624–6.
2. Kass EH. History of the specialty of infectious diseases in the United States. Ann Int Med 1987;106:745–56.

Preface

Vascular Medicine for Internists, Family Physicians, and Advanced Practice Providers

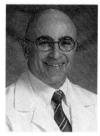 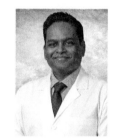

Geno J. Merli, MD, MACP, FSVM, FHM   Raghu Kolluri, MD, MS, RVT
Editors

Internal Medicine, Family Medicine, and Advanced Practice Providers frequently encounter patients who present with vascular disorders of the venous, arterial, and lymphatic circulations. These disorders manifest in a variety of symptoms and signs, which are important to recognize, assess, and treat. This issue of *Medical Clinics of North America* is devoted to the common vascular disorders experienced in practice.

The initial articles cover the pathogenesis of atherosclerotic vascular diseases, the assessment and management of peripheral arterial disease, and surgical interventions. Complementing these articles is a review of vascular imaging of the arterial and venous systems, which will aid in formulating a plan of management. Vasculitis and vasospastic disorders are reviewed to better understand the pathophysiology, assessment, and treatment of these disorders.

The remaining articles focus on venous diseases, which include varicose veins, venous thromboembolism management, approaches to unprovoked venous thrombosis, and engaging transitions of care for more effectively caring for this patient population.

Med Clin N Am 107 (2023) xvii–xviii
https://doi.org/10.1016/j.mcna.2023.05.010
0025-7125/23/© 2023 Published by Elsevier Inc.   medical.theclinics.com

The issue ends with a primer on approaching the patient with noncardiac lower-extremity swelling, which is a challenging situation faced by Internists and Family Physicians as well as Advanced Practice Providers.

Geno J. Merli, MD, MACP, FSVM, FHM
Division of Vascular Medicine
Sidney Kimmel Medical College
Thomas Jefferson University Hospitals
Jefferson Vascular Center
Suite 6210, Gibbon Building
111 South 11th Street
Philadelphia, PA 19107, USA

Raghu Kolluri, MD, MS, RVT
Vascular Medicine & Vascular Laboratories
OhioHealth Heart & Vascular
Ohio University HCOM
3705 Olentangy River Road, Suite 100
Columbus, OH 43214, USA

E-mail addresses:
geno.merli@jefferson.edu (G.J. Merli)
Kolluri.raghu@gmail.com (R. Kolluri)

Atherosclerotic Disease
Pathogenesis and Approaches to Management

Amanda M. Morrison, MD[a], Alexander E. Sullivan, MD[a],
Aaron W. Aday, MD, MSc[b],*

KEYWORDS

- Atherosclerosis • Smoking • Inflammation • Statins • Antiplatelet therapy

KEY POINTS

- Atherosclerosis is a complex, multifaceted process that is impacted by behavior, environment, genetics, and comorbid disease states.
- Inflammation represents a key pathophysiologic mechanism in the development and propagation of plaque formation.
- Management of atherosclerotic disease is multifaceted. Optimizing lifestyle through smoking cessation, diet, and exercise while concurrently optimizing medical therapies for hypertension, diabetes, and dyslipidemia is the cornerstone of mitigating cardiovascular risk.

BACKGROUND
Defining Atherosclerotic Disease

Atherosclerosis refers to the process of fibrofatty plaque formation within arterial walls. This process may lead to a hemodynamically significant narrowing and disruption of arterial flow to end-organs, manifesting as atherosclerotic disease.[1] Atherosclerosis may develop in any arterial segment and commonly leads to disease states in the coronary, carotid, cerebral, mesenteric, renal, and lower extremity arterial beds. Clinically, atherosclerosis in these distributions leads to important entities such as stroke, myocardial infarction (MI), coronary artery disease (CAD), mesenteric ischemia or ischemic colitis, and lower extremity peripheral artery disease (PAD). The risk of developing atherosclerotic disease is influenced by comorbidities, including dyslipidemia, hypertension, obesity, and diabetes. Management of these diseases may vary based on the clinical scenario and is aimed at mitigating or disrupting common pathways for

[a] Division of Cardiovascular Medicine, Department of Medicine, Vanderbilt University Medical Center, 1161 21st Avenue South, Nashville, TN 37232, USA; [b] Division of Cardiovascular Medicine, Department of Medicine, Vanderbilt Translational and Clinical Cardiovascular Research Center, Vanderbilt University Medical Center, 2525 West End Avenue, Suite 300, Nashville, TN 37203, USA
* Corresponding author.
E-mail address: aaron.w.aday@vumc.org

Med Clin N Am 107 (2023) 793–805
https://doi.org/10.1016/j.mcna.2023.04.004
medical.theclinics.com

the development of atherosclerosis. This article reviews the pathogenesis of athero-sclerotic disease as well as current approaches to managing patients with clinically stable atherosclerotic disease.

Impact of Atherosclerotic Disease

Collectively, atherosclerotic diseases represent the leading causes of death world-wide.[2] Stroke leads to one in six deaths, whereas the prevalence of CAD among adult Americans is estimated at 7.1% or around 20 million people. The prevalence of PAD is increasing and is now estimated to affect more than 236 million people worldwide.[3] An increasingly recognized clinical entity is polyvascular disease or atherosclerosis affecting multiple arterial beds, which increases the risk of future heart attack, stroke, or death.[4]

PATHOGENESIS OF PLAQUE FORMATION AND PROGRESSION
Mechanism of Plaque Formation

Arterial walls consist of three distinct layers, each having a unique role in maintaining vessel wall integrity and function. The adventitia is the outermost layer and contains the small blood vessels that feed the arterial wall (vasa vasorum), whereas smooth muscle cells and extracellular matrix proteins make up the media or middle layer.[5] The intima represents the innermost layer of the arterial wall and is lined with endothe-lial cells; the subendothelial space is the primary site of plaque formation. Plaque development occurs due to an interplay between endothelial cells, smooth muscle cells, and immune cells, including monocytes and macrophages (**Table 1**).[6] Vulnerable sections of endothelium develop in areas of turbulent or disrupted blood flow, commonly at sites of bifurcation, due to excessive hemodynamic stress.[7] This leads to increased endothelial permeability and activation of signaling molecules, including inflammatory mediators and cell adhesion molecules. Circulating lipoproteins, including low-density lipoprotein (LDL) particles, can traverse the endothelial layer

Table 1	
Key contributors in atherosclerotic plaque formation	
Key Players	**Role in Plaque Formation**
Endothelial cells	Activation under conditions of inflammation or stress, expression of adhesion molecules
Smooth muscle cells	Migration to the intimal layer, accumulation of extracellular matrix
Leukocyte adhesion molecules	Adherence of circulating monocytes and lymphocytes
Monocytes	Development of foam cells due to lipid uptake
Lymphocytes	Expression of pro-inflammatory mediators
Cytokines	Cell–cell communication; attract monocytes and macrophages
Platelet-derived growth factor	Promotes smooth muscle cell migration and proliferation, enhances extracellular matrix production
Interleukins (IL-1, IL-6)	Lymphocyte activation, innate immunity
Tumor necrosis factor	Leukocyte activation, cytokine release, production of reactive oxidative species
Colony-stimulating factor	Macrophage proliferation and survival
Interferon (IFN-γ)	Activation of monocytes, promotes formation of foam cells

Adapted from Libby P. The changing landscape of atherosclerosis. *Nature*. 2021;592(7855):524-533.

and become trapped in the subendothelial space, where they undergo oxidative changes that reinforce the local inflammatory response.[8] Reactive monocytes mature into macrophages as they are recruited to the intimal layer via attractant chemokines and activated platelets aggregate and adhere to the endothelium.[6] Foam cells form as mature macrophages attempt to clear oxidized lipoproteins via phagocytosis and ultimately undergo necrosis. The resulting cycle of localized chronic inflammation leads to the deposition of cell-breakdown products as well as fibrinous material deposited by smooth muscle cells attracted from the media into the intimal layer, which may propagate and extend into the vessel lumen as plaque.[5]

Plaque Histology

Plaque formation begins as fatty streaks or xanthomas, which are the result of lipid-rich foam cell aggregation within the intimal layer.[7] In response, smooth muscle cells proliferate and migrate from the media to intima, leading to intimal hyperplasia.[1] As this process continues, the smooth muscle cells organize and deposit extracellular matrix, forming a fibrous cap.[9] If this process is uninterrupted, the plaque continues to proliferate and enlarge, ultimately producing a hemodynamically significant stenosis. Erosion or rupture of the fibrous cap can lead to thrombotic occlusion or distal embolism due to exposure of bloodstream coagulation factors with thrombogenic plaque material, causing platelet aggregation, obstruction of blood flow, and resultant end-organ ischemia.[10,11] Several features have historically defined plaque vulnerability or propensity to rupture (**Table 2**). Lesions with these findings are at greater risk of causing a future vascular event.[9]

RISK FACTORS FOR ATHEROSCLEROSIS DEVELOPMENT
Smoking

Cigarette smoking remains one of the leading preventable risk factors for the development of atherosclerotic disease. The prevalence of cigarette smoking daily or some days for adults in the United States is estimated at 14%.[2] Overall rates of cigarette smoking have declined significantly in recent decades, but former smokers remain at excess risk for atherosclerotic disease.[2] Cigarette smoking likely perpetuates the cycle of local inflammation, endothelial damage, and pro-thrombotic conditions that lead to atherosclerosis, but these mechanisms are incompletely understood.[12]

Diet

Dietary patterns contribute to the development of atherosclerosis through alterations in blood pressure (BP), circulating lipoprotein concentrations, insulin resistance, inflammation, and oxidative stress.[13] Emerging evidence suggests that overall diet

Table 2
Histopathologic features of stable and vulnerable plaques

Vulnerable Plaque	Stable Plaque
Thin fibrous cap	Thick fibrous cap
Large lipid-rich and/or necrotic core	Small lipid core without necrosis
Intraplaque hemorrhage	Plaque calcification
Plaque ulceration	Smooth plaque
Local inflammation	Absence of significant inflammation

Risk of plaque rupture increases in the setting of vulnerable plaque.[10]

quality, rather than specific food groups, leads to changes in the gut microbiome, hepatic lipogenesis, and metabolism.[13] Poor dietary quality, especially when combined with a sedentary lifestyle, predisposes patients to higher rates of obesity and metabolic syndrome and subsequent increased atherosclerotic risk.[2]

Obesity

Obesity is associated with the development of atherosclerotic disease and is linked to increases in circulating lipoproteins, including LDL and triglycerides.[2,14] Excess adipose tissue releases signaling molecules that increase systemic inflammation, enhance hypercoagulability, worsen insulin resistance, and promote endothelial dysfunction.[15]

Dyslipidemia

Elevated blood concentration of LDL cholesterol (LDL-C) in humans is causally linked to atherosclerotic disease.[16] Pro-inflammatory and pro-immunogenic properties of oxidized LDL underlie this relationship, though more recent studies have questioned the role of oxidized LDL.[11,17] In recent years, there has been increasing interest in triglyceride-rich lipoproteins, which are pro-atherogenic and pro-inflammatory,[18] as well as blood elevations in lipoprotein (a) (Lp[a]).[19]

Hypertension

Elevated BP is associated with increased atherosclerotic disease risk, primarily driven by increases in shear stress along the vascular endothelial surface, arteriolar remodeling, vascular stiffness, and dysregulated cellular sodium processing.[20] Lymphocytes and monocyte/macrophages accumulate within perivascular renal arterioles in response to chronically elevated BP and release cytokines that enhance oxidative stress, immune activation, and vascular dysfunction.[21]

Diabetes

Diabetes and insulin resistance have well-documented associations with atherosclerosis and cardiovascular risk.[22] Hyperinsulinemia causes increases in circulating fatty acids, which are pro-inflammatory and pro-atherogenic.[18] Excess circulating glucose leads to glycosylation of enzymes which may increase oxidative stress and enhance pro-inflammatory pathways.[23] These factors collectively lead to modification of the microvascular and macrovascular structure and promote the formation and progression of plaque.[21,23]

INFLAMMATION

Local inflammation drives plaque propagation, erosion, and rupture and may be the common pathway by which many traditional risk factors lead to atherosclerosis. Systemic inflammation can be initiated by excess circulating fatty acid intermediates, glycosylated lipoprotein products, or hypertension, ultimately leading to alterations in circulating immune cells and increases in oxidative stress.[23] Inflammasomes, or large intracellular multimeric protein complexes activated in response to local tissue damage, are thought to drive this inflammatory response by controlling the release of inflammatory cytokines, including interleukin (IL)-1β and IL-18.[21,24] These cytokines are elevated in disease states including CAD and lead to downstream expression of systemic inflammatory mediators including tumor necrosis factor and IL-6.[24] The role of novel anti-inflammatory therapies, including those targeting IL-1β and IL-6, in mitigating future cardiovascular risk remains an area of active research.[25]

THROMBOSIS

Arterial thrombosis is the eventual mechanism by which obstruction of blood flow occurs in atherosclerotic disease. Local thrombosis occurs due to rupture or erosion of plaque and exposure of necrotic or lipid-rich core components to the systemic circulation, which results in platelet aggregation, platelet activation, and induction of the coagulation cascade via tissue factor release.[26] Platelet-rich thrombi form and ultimately lead to vessel occlusion if uninhibited.[26] In addition to lipid-lowering therapies, pharmacotherapy to interrupt or prevent the thrombotic process is a mainstay of management.

MANAGEMENT OF STABLE ATHEROSCLEROTIC DISEASE

Atherosclerosis requires a multifaceted management approach that needs to be tailored to the individual patient risk profile. The astute clinician must identify opportunities for risk reduction and dynamically tailor therapies throughout years of management.

Smoking Cessation

In heavy smokers, cessation is associated with a nearly 40% reduction in cardiovascular risk within 5 years, but the cardiovascular risk remains elevated compared with never-smokers for up to 25 years after cessation.[27] Many patients struggle with tobacco cessation, and fewer than 10% of patients who attempt to quit are successful. Referral to a multidisciplinary smoking cessation program that includes pharmacotherapy and behavioral intervention increases the likelihood of achieving abstinence threefold and should be the cornerstone of management.[28] Varenicline, nicotine replacement therapy (NRT), and bupropion are well-established therapies recommended for cessation by multiple societal guidelines and consensus statements.[29] Varenicline is superior to both NRT and bupropion in 6-month tobacco abstinence and has even greater efficacy when combined with long- and short-acting NRT.[30] NRT is most effective when prescribed in both long- and short-acting formulations to provide both basal and bolus coverage.

Diet and Exercise

A healthy diet and physical activity are key components of atherosclerotic prevention, particularly as obesity rates rise across the United States.[31] Societal guidelines recommend counseling patients at every visit on the importance of a diet rich in vegetables, fruits, nuts, whole grains, lean animal protein, and fish while minimizing *trans* fats, red and processed meats, refined carbohydrates, and sweetened beverages.[32] Although not directly linked to atherosclerosis, diets high in sodium (>2000 mg daily) have been linked to increased BP and increased risk of cardiovascular events.[33] Although large-scale randomized controlled trials with hard cardiovascular endpoints are limited, multiple observational studies have demonstrated an association between poor dietary habits and cardiovascular mortality.[32]

Physical activity offers several beneficial cardiovascular effects, including improved physical functioning, weight reduction, and glycemic and BP control.[32] There is a strong, inverse, dose–response relationship between physical activity and cardiovascular events, and current guidelines recommend at least 150 minutes per week of accumulated moderate-intensity physical activity or 75 minutes per week of vigorous-intensity physical activity.[33] Patients should be regularly counseled on the benefits of an active lifestyle, especially those with established atherosclerotic disease, obesity, or diabetes mellitus who are at greatest cardiovascular risk.[34]

Blood Pressure Control

Nearly 50% of Americans meet the criteria for hypertension and approximately 25% are on antihypertensive medications.[35] Each 20 mm Hg rise in systolic BP (SBP) above 115 and 10 mm Hg rise in diastolic BP (DBP) above 75 mm Hg is associated with a twofold increase in risk of death from stroke, heart disease, or other atherosclerotic vascular diseases.[36] Patients with atherosclerotic disease should be treated to BP targets of SBP less than 130 mm Hg and DBP less than 80 mm Hg, as intensive BP control is associated with significant reductions in cardiovascular events, even in elderly patients.[37] All patients with atherosclerosis should be started on pharmacologic therapy if not at goal. American College of Cardiology/American Heart Association guidelines recommend combination therapy for Black patients and for adults with more severe hypertension (SBP$\geq$140 mm Hg or DBP $\geq$90 mm Hg and an average SBP/DBP >20/10 mm Hg above their target BP).[37] Calcium channel blockers, thiazide diuretics, angiotensin-converting-enzyme inhibitors (ACEi), or angiotensin receptor blockers (ARBs) should be used as initial pharmacologic agents and selected based on the patient profile (**Table 3**).[37]

Glycemic Control

Lifestyle modification (as described above) should be discussed at every preventative health visit to reduce the risk of developing metabolic syndrome and type 2 diabetes mellitus (T2DM). When this has failed, the American Diabetes Association recommends a hemoglobin A1c target of less than 7% for most nonpregnant adults, less than 6.5% for young patients, and less than 8% for those with limited life expectancy.[38] Intensification of lifestyle modification remains first-line therapy to improve glycemic control. This includes dietary modification, such as adhering to a Mediterranean, dietary approaches to stop hypertension (DASH), or vegetarian/vegan diet, institution of an exercise program, and weight loss.[32] Metformin is the first-line choice once pharmacologic therapy is needed and has beneficial effects on hyperglycemia, weight loss, and atherosclerotic risk.[32] In those with additional risk factors for atherosclerotic disease, sodium-glucose cotransporter-2 (SGLT-2) inhibitors and glucagon-like peptide-1 receptor agonists have been shown to significantly reduce cardiovascular events and can be added to metformin if additional glycemic control is needed.[39,40] SGLT-2 inhibitors should be preferentially selected for patients with atherosclerosis and T2DM who also have concurrent heart failure or albuminuria.[41]

Lipid-Lowering Therapies

Statins reduce LDL-C levels and risk of cardiovascular disease in those with atherosclerotic disease and are the preferred initial therapy for hyperlipidemia (**Table 4**).[42,43] Goal LDL-C reduction is $\geq$ 50% or to a target of $\leq$ 70 mg/dL for those at high risk, which includes all patients with prior atherosclerotic cardiovascular events.[44] Those patients with established atherosclerotic disease but without prior cardiovascular events should be stratified by atherosclerotic cardiovascular disease risk score, and any recommendation for moderate versus high-intensity statin should be based on those results.[44] For patients not at goal with high-intensity statin therapy alone, ezetimibe is the most commonly used non-statin therapy and lowers LDL-C by an additional 13% to 20%.[44] Proprotein convertase subtilisin/kexin type 9 (PCSK9) inhibitors are powerful LDL-lowing drugs that reduce LDL-C levels by 43% to 64% and have been shown to reduce atherosclerotic risk in patients not achieving LDL-C goal with maximally tolerated statin therapy and ezetimibe. Ongoing studies are testing the

Table 3
Antihypertensive therapy

Therapy	Dose	Prescribing Considerations
ACEi or ARB[a]	Usual dosing range: ACEi: Benazepril 10–40 mg/d (1–2 doses) Captopril 12.5–150 mg/d (2–3 doses) Enalapril 5–40 mg/d (1–2 doses) Lisinopril 10–40 mg/d (1 dose) Usual dosing range: ARB: Candesartan 8–32 mg/d (1 dose) Irbesartan 150–300 mg/d (1 dose) Losartan 50–100 mg/d(1–2 doses) Valsartan 80–320 mg/d (1 doses)	Use in patients with DM, HF, microalbuminuria Consider combination use with thiazide diuretic or CCB Monitor eGFR and potassium after initiation Avoid monotherapy in black patients unless additional indication Avoid combination of ACEi/ARB/direct renin inhibitors
CCB[a]	Usual dosing range: Amlodipine 2.5–10 mg/d (1 dose) Nifedipine SR 60–120 mg/d (2 doses) Nifedipine LA 30–90 mg/d (1 dose)	Avoid in HF Monitor for lower extremity edema Thiazide diuretic or CCB preferred first line in black adults without HF or CKD (even if DM present).
Thiazide diuretic[a]	Usual dosing range: Chlorthalidone 12.5–25 mg/d (1 dose) Hydrochlorothiazide 25–50 mg/d (1 dose)	Monitor for hyponatremia and hypokalemia, and calcium levels.
MRAs	Usual dosing range: Eplerenone 50–100 mg/d (1–2 doses) Spironolactone 25–100 mg/d (1 dose)	Fourth-line agent Monitor for hyperkalemia

Abbreviations: ACEi, angiotensin-converting enzyme inhibitors; ARB, angiotensin receptor blockers; CCB, calcium channel blocker; CKD, chronic kidney disease; d, day; DM, diabetes mellitus; eGFR, estimated glomerular filtration rate; HF, heart failure; mg, milligram; MRA, mineralocorticoid receptor antagonist.
[a] First line.

Table 4
Lipid-lowering therapy

Therapy	Dose	Prescribing Considerations
Statin	Usual dosing range: High intensity: Atorvastatin 40–80 mg/d Rosuvastatin 20–40 mg/d Usual dosing range: Moderate intensity: Atorvastatin 10–20 mg/d Rosuvastatin 5–10 mg/d Simvastatin 20–40 mg/d Pravastatin 40–80 mg/d Lovastatin 40–80 mg/d Fluvastatin 80 mg/d	Monitor for subjective myalgias (5%–20% of patients) Rhabdomyolysis and hepatotoxicity rare but serious complications
Ezetimibe[59]	Usual dosing range: Ezetimibe 10 mg/d	Up to 20% LDL-C reduction Generally well tolerated
PCSK9 inhibitors	Usual dosing range: PCSK9 antibodies: Alirocumab[60] • Initial: 75 mg/2 wk or 300 mg/4 wk • Max: 150 mg/2 wk Evolucumab[61] • 140 mg/2 wk or 420 mg/mo	Subcutaneous administration Side effects: flu-like symptoms, injection site reactions, muscle aches

Abbreviations: d, day; LDL-C, low-density lipoprotein cholesterol; mg, milligram; PCSK9, proprotein convertase subtilisin/kexin type 9.

efficacy of small interfering RNA (siRNA) molecules to achieve long-term LDL or Lp(a) reduction.[45]

Antiplatelet Therapy

Aspirin has been widely used for the prevention of atherosclerotic events. In patients who have had a prior MI, transient ischemic attack (TIA), or stroke, aspirin is a mainstay of secondary prevention, and extensive data support its use to reduce atherosclerotic events.[46]

P2Y$_{12}$ inhibitors, such as clopidogrel, ticagrelor, and prasugrel, are more potent and efficacious antiplatelet agents.[47] These agents are commonly used in combination with aspirin (termed dual antiplatelet therapy [DAPT]) for the prevention of ischemic events following acute coronary syndrome, percutaneous coronary intervention, and TIA/stroke.[48,49] Duration of therapy following an acute event depends on the clinical syndrome and patient profile. Antiplatelet regimens should be tailored to the individual patient's bleeding and ischemic risk while also considering the location of atherosclerosis and prior procedural characteristics that may increase the risk of future cardiovascular events. In patients with stable atherosclerotic disease, there is evidence that chronic P2Y$_{12}$ inhibitor monotherapy may be more efficacious than aspirin without incurring a higher risk of bleeding.[50]

Antithrombotic Therapy

Antithrombotic therapy plays an important role in reducing long-term cardiovascular risk in individuals with atherosclerotic disease, particularly those with polyvascular disease. The Cardiovascular Outcomes for People Using Anticoagulation Strategies trial found that rivaroxaban 2.5 mg daily in combination with aspirin reduced the composite event of cardiovascular death, MI, and stroke compared with aspirin alone in patients with CAD and PAD.[51] Similar results were seen in subgroup analyses of patients with PAD with additional reductions in major adverse limb events.[52] A subsequent trial also demonstrated a reduction in acute limb ischemia, major amputation, MI, ischemic stroke, and cardiovascular death with rivaroxaban 2.5 mg twice daily and aspirin compared with aspirin alone in patients undergoing lower extremity revascularization.[53] Rivaroxaban 2.5 mg twice daily with low-dose aspirin should be considered in all patients with stable atherosclerotic disease in $\geq$ 2 vascular beds and acceptable bleeding risk.

Clinics Care Points: Antiplatelet and Antithrombotic Therapy in Polyvascular Disease

- Pearls
  - Identification of polyvascular disease is the first step in determining appropriate management.
  - Common definitions:
    - CAD: stenosis $\geq$50%, prior percutaneous coronary intervention, or prior coronary artery bypass graft surgery
    - PAD: Ankle-brachial index (ABI) less than 0.9 or $\geq$ 50% stenosis of lower extremity artery
    - Cerebrovascular disease (CVD): prior stroke, TIA, or $\geq$50% stenosis of carotid artery
  - Once individuals with polyvascular disease are identified, medical management varies by affected vascular bed.
- Pitfalls
  - Polyvascular disease is often overlooked, and clinicians may presume treatment of atherosclerosis does not vary by arterial distribution.
  - Even patients with atherosclerotic obstruction in an arterial bed but without obvious symptoms remain at heightened risk of cardiovascular events.
- Recommendations[50,54]
  - In patients with stable CAD, CVD, or PAD, aspirin is first line for risk reduction. Clopidogrel can be utilized as monotherapy in select patients, particularly those with PAD.
  - In patients with stable CAD and either CVD and/or PAD, aspirin should be combined with low-dose rivaroxaban.
  - Following any revascularization, DAPT is typically indicated, with the exception of lower extremity revascularization where aspirin, low-dose rivaroxaban, $\pm$ clopidogrel should be used.
  - Deescalation of therapy after an acute event should be tailored to the individual patient's bleeding and ischemic risk.

SUMMARY AND FUTURE DIRECTIONS

Despite a better understanding of risk factors and disease-modifying interventions, atherosclerosis continues to affect millions of people with significant ramification for the health care system. There are numerous ongoing efforts to identify novel risk factors, better calculate individual risk, and develop unique therapeutic interventions with the ultimate goal of further mitigating atherosclerotic disease burden. Newly appreciated risk factors, such as clonal hematopoiesis of indeterminate potential and air pollution, are linked to excess cardiovascular risk through pro-inflammatory or pro-thrombotic properties.[11,55] Advances in genomics are bringing personalized genetic risk assessment closer to a reality along with the possibility of genome editing as a therapeutic intervention.[56] Novel therapeutic drugs, namely siRNAs, have been developed which can dramatically reduce LDL-C or Lp(a) concentrations with only a few doses each year, and phase III trials of these drugs are ongoing.[57,58] Collectively, these areas of active research will dramatically impact our strategies for prevention and treatment of atherosclerosis in the near future.

DISCLOSURE

This work was supporting by the National Institutes of Health, United States T32 GM007569 (A.E. Sullivan) and K23 HL151871 (A.W. Aday). A.W. Aday reports receiving consulting fees from OptumCare, CRC Oncology, and Aeglea outside of the current work. All other authors report no conflicts.

REFERENCES

1. Chan YH, Ramji DP. Atherosclerosis: Pathogenesis and Key Cellular Processes, Current and Emerging Therapies, Key Challenges, and Future Research Directions. Methods Mol Biol 2022;2419:3–19.
2. Tsao CW, Aday AW, Almarzooq ZI, et al. Heart Disease and Stroke Statistics-2023 Update: A Report From the American Heart Association. Circulation 2023. https://doi.org/10.1161/CIR.0000000000001123.
3. Song P, Rudan D, Zhu Y, et al. Global, regional, and national prevalence and risk factors for peripheral artery disease in 2015: an updated systematic review and analysis. Lancet Glob Health 2019;7(8):e1020–30.
4. Aday AW, Matsushita K. Epidemiology of Peripheral Artery Disease and Polyvascular Disease. Circ Res 2021;128(12):1818–32.
5. Libby P, Buring JE, Badimon L, et al. Atherosclerosis. Nat Rev Dis Primers 2019; 5(1):56.
6. Ramji DP, Ismail A, Chen J, et al. Survey of In Vitro Model Systems for Investigation of Key Cellular Processes Associated with Atherosclerosis. Methods Mol Biol 2022;2419:39–56.
7. Franck G, Even G, Gautier A, et al. Haemodynamic stress-induced breaches of the arterial intima trigger inflammation and drive atherogenesis. Eur Heart J 2019;40(11):928–37.
8. Libby P, Hansson GK. From Focal Lipid Storage to Systemic Inflammation: JACC Review Topic of the Week. J Am Coll Cardiol 2019;74(12):1594–607.
9. Waksman R, Torguson R, Spad MA, et al. The Lipid-Rich Plaque Study of vulnerable plaques and vulnerable patients: Study design and rationale. Am Heart J 2017;192:98–104.
10. Hansson GK, Libby P, Tabas I. Inflammation and plaque vulnerability. J Intern Med 2015;278(5):483–93.
11. Libby P. The changing landscape of atherosclerosis. Nature 2021;592(7855): 524–33.
12. Messner B, Bernhard D. Smoking and cardiovascular disease: mechanisms of endothelial dysfunction and early atherogenesis. Arterioscler Thromb Vasc Biol 2014;34(3):509–15.
13. Mozaffarian D. Dietary and Policy Priorities for Cardiovascular Disease, Diabetes, and Obesity: A Comprehensive Review. Circulation 2016;133(2):187–225.
14. Falaschetti E, Hingorani AD, Jones A, et al. Adiposity and cardiovascular risk factors in a large contemporary population of pre-pubertal children. Eur Heart J 2010;31(24):3063–72.
15. Rocha VZ, Libby P. Obesity, inflammation, and atherosclerosis. Nat Rev Cardiol 2009;6(6):399–409.

16. Ference BA, Ginsberg HN, Graham I, et al. Low-density lipoproteins cause atherosclerotic cardiovascular disease. 1. Evidence from genetic, epidemiologic, and clinical studies. A consensus statement from the European Atherosclerosis Society Consensus Panel. Eur Heart J 2017;38(32):2459–72.
17. Navab M, Ananthramaiah GM, Reddy ST, et al. The oxidation hypothesis of atherogenesis: the role of oxidized phospholipids and HDL. J Lipid Res 2004; 45(6):993–1007.
18. Nordestgaard BG. Triglyceride-Rich Lipoproteins and Atherosclerotic Cardiovascular Disease: New Insights From Epidemiology, Genetics, and Biology. Circ Res 2016;118(4):547–63.
19. Burgess S, Ference BA, Staley JR, et al. Association of LPA Variants With Risk of Coronary Disease and the Implications for Lipoprotein(a)-Lowering Therapies: A Mendelian Randomization Analysis. JAMA Cardiol 2018;3(7):619–27.
20. Safar ME, Levy BI, Struijker-Boudier H. Current perspectives on arterial stiffness and pulse pressure in hypertension and cardiovascular diseases. Circulation 2003;107(22):2864–9.
21. McMaster WG, Kirabo A, Madhur MS, et al. Inflammation, immunity, and hypertensive end-organ damage. Circ Res 2015;116(6):1022–33.
22. Stratton IM, Adler AI, Neil HA, et al. Association of glycaemia with macrovascular and microvascular complications of type 2 diabetes (UKPDS 35): prospective observational study. BMJ 2000;321(7258):405–12.
23. Libby P, Plutzky J. Diabetic macrovascular disease: the glucose paradox? Circulation 2002;106(22):2760–3.
24. Olsen MB, Gregersen I, Sandanger Ø, et al. Targeting the Inflammasome in Cardiovascular Disease. JACC Basic Transl Sci 2022;7(1):84–98.
25. Soehnlein O, Libby P. Targeting inflammation in atherosclerosis - from experimental insights to the clinic. Nat Rev Drug Discov 2021;20(8):589–610.
26. Mackman N. Triggers, targets and treatments for thrombosis. Nature 2008; 451(7181):914–8.
27. Duncan MS, Freiberg MS, Greevy RA Jr, et al. Association of Smoking Cessation With Subsequent Risk of Cardiovascular Disease. JAMA 2019;322(7):642–50.
28. Hennrikus D, Joseph AM, Lando HA, et al. Effectiveness of a smoking cessation program for peripheral artery disease patients: a randomized controlled trial. J Am Coll Cardiol 2010;56(25):2105–12.
29. Barua RS, Rigotti NA, Benowitz NL, et al. 2018 ACC Expert Consensus Decision Pathway on Tobacco Cessation Treatment: A Report of the American College of Cardiology Task Force on Clinical Expert Consensus Documents. J Am Coll Cardiol 2018;72(25):3332–65.
30. Patnode CD, Henderson JT, Coppola EL, et al. Interventions for Tobacco Cessation in Adults, Including Pregnant Persons: Updated Evidence Report and Systematic Review for the US Preventive Services Task Force. JAMA 2021;325(3): 280–98.
31. Ward ZJ, Bleich SN, Cradock AL, et al. Projected U.S. State-Level Prevalence of Adult Obesity and Severe Obesity. N Engl J Med 2019;381(25):2440–50.
32. Arnett DK, Blumenthal RS, Albert MA, et al. 2019 ACC/AHA Guideline on the Primary Prevention of Cardiovascular Disease: Executive Summary: A Report of the American College of Cardiology/American Heart Association Task Force on Clinical Practice Guidelines. J Am Coll Cardiol 2019;74(10):1376–414.
33. Cook NR, Cutler JA, Obarzanek E, et al. Long term effects of dietary sodium reduction on cardiovascular disease outcomes: observational follow-up of the trials of hypertension prevention (TOHP). BMJ 2007;334(7599):885–8.

34. Sluik D, Buijsse B, Muckelbauer R, et al. Physical Activity and Mortality in Individuals With Diabetes Mellitus: A Prospective Study and Meta-analysis. Arch Intern Med 2012;172(17):1285–95.

35. Muntner P, Carey RM, Gidding S, et al. Potential US Population Impact of the 2017 ACC/AHA High Blood Pressure Guideline. Circulation 2018;137(2):109–18.

36. Lewington S, Clarke R, Qizilbash N, et al. Age-specific relevance of usual blood pressure to vascular mortality: a meta-analysis of individual data for one million adults in 61 prospective studies. Lancet 2002;360(9349):1903–13.

37. Whelton PK, Carey RM, Aronow WS, et al. 2017 ACC/AHA/AAPA/ABC/ACPM/AGS/APhA/ASH/ASPC/NMA/PCNA Guideline for the Prevention, Detection, Evaluation, and Management of High Blood Pressure in Adults: A Report of the American College of Cardiology/American Heart Association Task Force on Clinical Practice Guidelines. J Am Coll Cardiol 2018;71(19):e127–248.

38. Joseph JJ, Deedwania P, Acharya T, et al. Comprehensive Management of Cardiovascular Risk Factors for Adults With Type 2 Diabetes: A Scientific Statement From the American Heart Association. Circulation 2022;145(9):e722–59.

39. Marso SP, Daniels GH, Brown-Frandsen K, et al. Liraglutide and Cardiovascular Outcomes in Type 2 Diabetes. N Engl J Med 2016;375(4):311–22.

40. Zinman B, Wanner C, Lachin JM, et al. Empagliflozin, Cardiovascular Outcomes, and Mortality in Type 2 Diabetes. N Engl J Med 2015;373(22):2117–28.

41. Solis-Herrera C, Cersosimo E, Triplitt C. Antihyperglycemic Algorithms for Type 2 Diabetes: Focus on Nonglycemic Outcomes. Diabetes Spectr 2021;34(3):248–56.

42. Amarenco P, Bogousslavsky J, Callahan A 3rd, et al. High-dose atorvastatin after stroke or transient ischemic attack. N Engl J Med 2006;355(6):549–59.

43. Ridker PM, Danielson E, Fonseca FA, et al. Rosuvastatin to prevent vascular events in men and women with elevated C-reactive protein. N Engl J Med 2008;359(21):2195–207.

44. Grundy SM, Stone NJ, Bailey AL, et al. 2018 AHA/ACC/AACVPR/AAPA/ABC/ACPM/ADA/AGS/APhA/ASPC/NLA/PCNA Guideline on the Management of Blood Cholesterol: Executive Summary: A Report of the American College of Cardiology/American Heart Association Task Force on Clinical Practice Guidelines. Circulation 2019;139(25):e1046–81.

45. Ray KK, Stoekenbroek RM, Kallend D, et al. Effect of an siRNA Therapeutic Targeting PCSK9 on Atherogenic Lipoproteins: Prespecified Secondary End Points in ORION 1. Circulation 2018;138(13):1304–16.

46. Baigent C, Blackwell L, Collins R, et al. Aspirin in the primary and secondary prevention of vascular disease: collaborative meta-analysis of individual participant data from randomised trials. Lancet 2009;373(9678):1849–60.

47. Aggarwal D, Bhatia K, Chunawala ZS, et al. P2Y(12) inhibitor versus aspirin monotherapy for secondary prevention of cardiovascular events: meta-analysis of randomized trials. Eur Heart J Open 2022;2(2):oeac019.

48. Yusuf S, Zhao F, Mehta SR, et al. Effects of clopidogrel in addition to aspirin in patients with acute coronary syndromes without ST-segment elevation. N Engl J Med 2001;345(7):494–502.

49. Johnston SC, Easton JD, Farrant M, et al. Clopidogrel and Aspirin in Acute Ischemic Stroke and High-Risk TIA. N Engl J Med 2018;379(3):215–25.

50. A randomised, blinded, trial of clopidogrel versus aspirin in patients at risk of ischaemic events (CAPRIE). CAPRIE Steering Committee. Lancet 1996;348(9038):1329–39.

51. Eikelboom JW, Connolly SJ, Bosch J, et al. Rivaroxaban with or without Aspirin in Stable Cardiovascular Disease. N Engl J Med 2017;377(14):1319–30.
52. Anand SS, Bosch J, Eikelboom JW, et al. Rivaroxaban with or without aspirin in patients with stable peripheral or carotid artery disease: an international, randomised, double-blind, placebo-controlled trial. Lancet 2018;391(10117):219–29.
53. Bonaca MP, Bauersachs RM, Anand SS, et al. Rivaroxaban in Peripheral Artery Disease after Revascularization. N Engl J Med 2020;382(21):1994–2004.
54. Hess CN, Hiatt WR. Antithrombotic Therapy for Peripheral Artery Disease in 2018. JAMA 2018;319(22):2329–30.
55. Jaiswal S, Natarajan P, Silver AJ, et al. Clonal Hematopoiesis and Risk of Atherosclerotic Cardiovascular Disease. N Engl J Med 2017;377(2):111–21.
56. Seeger T, Porteus M, Wu JC. Genome Editing in Cardiovascular Biology. Circ Res 2017;120(5):778–80.
57. Ray KK, Wright RS, Kallend D, et al. Two Phase 3 Trials of Inclisiran in Patients with Elevated LDL Cholesterol. N Engl J Med 2020;382(16):1507–19.
58. O'Donoghue ML, Rosenson RS, Gencer B, et al. Small Interfering RNA to Reduce Lipoprotein(a) in Cardiovascular Disease. N Engl J Med 2022;387(20):1855–64.
59. Cannon CP, Blazing MA, Giugliano RP, et al. Ezetimibe Added to Statin Therapy after Acute Coronary Syndromes. N Engl J Med 2015;372(25):2387–97.
60. Schwartz GG, Steg PG, Szarek M, et al. Alirocumab and Cardiovascular Outcomes after Acute Coronary Syndrome. N Engl J Med 2018;379(22):2097–107.
61. Sabatine MS, Giugliano RP, Keech AC, et al. Evolocumab and Clinical Outcomes in Patients with Cardiovascular Disease. N Engl J Med 2017;376(18):1713–22.

Peripheral Artery Disease
Overview of Diagnosis and Medical Therapy

Matthew Bierowski, MD[a], Taki Galanis, MD[b,*],
Amry Majeed, MD[a], Alireza Mofid, MD[c]

KEYWORDS

- Peripheral artery disease • Claudication • Ankle-brachial index • Limb ischemia

KEY POINTS

- Peripheral artery disease (PAD) is very common and affects approximately 230 and 5 million people worldwide and nationally, respectively.
- Race and socioeconomic status have profound impacts on PAD outcomes.
- PAD is an underrecognized and undertreated medical condition.

EPIDEMIOLOGY

The worldwide prevalence of peripheral artery disease (PAD) is estimated to be 5% with approximately 230 million people affected by this disease globally.[1] In the United States, at least 5 million people are impacted by this condition, as per the National Health and Nutrition Examination Survey conducted from 1999 to 2004. Within that cohort, PAD prevalence was significantly higher among those with low income and lower levels of education.[2] Specifically, those in the lowest income group had a greater than a twofold increased odds of PAD compared with the highest income group. Globally, low- and middle-income regions saw a near 30% increase in PAD from 2000 to 2010 compared with a 13% increase in high-income regions.[3]

Racial disparities also exist with a higher prevalence among black men when compared with non-Hispanic and Caucasian men.[4] Prevalence was similar between Hispanic, American Indian, and Caucasian men. Of note, Asian men had the lowest prevalence. Such trends were similar among women, other than Indian American women having similar prevalence to black women.[4] The overall lifetime estimate of PAD is 20% for Caucasians and 30% for black patients.[5]

[a] Internal Medicine, Thomas Jefferson University Hospital, 1025 Walnut Street, Philadelphia, PA 19107, USA; [b] Division Vascular Medicine, Jefferson Vascular Center, Sidney Kimmel Medical College, Philadelphia, PA, USA; [c] Vascular Surgery, Thomas Jefferson University Hospital, 111 South 11th Street, Suite 6210 Gibbon, Philadelphia, PA 19107, USA
* Corresponding author. 111 South 11th Street, Suite 6210 Gibbon, Philadelphia, PA 19107.
E-mail address: Taki.Galanis@jefferson.edu

Med Clin N Am 107 (2023) 807–822
https://doi.org/10.1016/j.mcna.2023.05.007

- PAD is very common and affects approximately 230 and 5 million people world-wide and nationally, respectively.
- There is a higher prevalence of PAD in black patients, with an overall lifetime estimate of 30% for these individuals compared with 20% for Caucasians.

RISK FACTORS

Risk factors associated with the development of PAD are like its counterpart, coronary artery disease (CAD). Such risk factors include age, family history, socioeconomic status (SES), tobacco smoking, diabetes mellitus, and hypertension (systolic pressure).[2,4,6–9] Neither sex[10,11] nor low-density lipoprotein (LDL) levels[12,13] have consistently correlated to an increased risk of PAD. However, multiple studies have found a link between high-density lipoprotein (HDL) levels and total cholesterol:HDL levels and PAD.[13–15] Of note, tobacco smoking is the strongest risk factor, followed closely by diabetes.[3]

The Scottish Heart Health Extended Cohort examined over 15,000 individuals aged 30 to 75 years who had either PAD or CAD, but not both, and followed the participants for 15 to 25 years. Although many of the risk factors discussed above overlapped between the two conditions, in the PAD population, tobacco smoking and inflammatory markers dominated, whereas cholesterol levels and body mass index (BMI) were less consistent risk factors. Specifically, increasing age, C-reactive protein levels, tobacco smoking, systolic blood pressure, and SES delegated the highest hazard ratios for PAD.[16]

Key Points

- The risk factors for PAD overlap for CAD. However, inflammatory markers, increasing age, and SES are associated with greater hazard ratios for PAD compared with CAD.
- Tobacco smoking is the strongest risk factor for PAD.

SOCIOECONOMIC AND RACIAL DISPARITIES

Although low SES has been linked with worse outcomes for CAD, diabetes, hypertension, and smoking, previously there was little research on SES and PAD outcomes. However, over the past few years, several studies have highlighted the negative impact on outcomes in PAD associated with low SES and race. Specifically, low SES was associated with higher rates of amputation not only across every race, but also within each subgroup of race (ie, diabetics, CKD).[17] Several studies have highlighted the vast disparities of PAD outcomes within metropolitan areas. Zip codes with lower SES were associated with higher amputation rates, even with adjustments for clinical and demographic factors.[18] Furthermore, within these low SES zip codes, black patients overwhelmingly account for the vast majority of these cases. Not surprisingly, zip codes associated with high numbers of black residents were associated with some of the highest amputation rates.[18] Black patients, on average, were two- to threefold more likely to have an amputation when admitted to the hospital with critical limb ischemia compared with their white counterparts.[19] Among Medicare beneficiaries, black patients were less likely than their white counterparts to be offered limb-salvaging procedures, likely due to a combination of more severe disease and racial biases in health care.[20] Black patients were also more likely to have higher incidences of femoral-tibial or popliteal-tibial bypass when compared with whites.[21] This is likely due to blacks, on average, having more severe PAD at the time of the initial diagnosis when compared with whites[20,22,23] and in part due to blacks having lower rates of prescriptions for statin and antiplatelet agents.[17]

Key Points

- Race and SES have profound impacts on PAD outcomes.
- Zip codes with low SES have the highest amputation rates.
- Black patients are more likely than Caucasians to undergo an amputation when admitted to the hospital and are less likely to be offered limb-salvaging procedures.

CLINICAL PRESENTATION AND DIAGNOSIS

The initial diagnosis of PAD remains a challenge for providers as nearly 50% of patients with PAD are unaware of their disease along with 30% of providers being unaware of their patients having PAD.[24] The clinical diagnosis is made even more challenging as only 10% of patients will present with classic intermittent claudication symptoms, whereas 50% will have atypical symptoms such as exertional lower extremity pain that does not resolve with rest or discomfort that does not consistently limit exercise at increasing distances. The remaining 40% will be asymptomatic.[25] A greater likelihood of atypical symptoms is likely due in part to the common comorbidities that accompany patients with PAD, such as arthritis, neuropathy, spinal canal pathology, fibromyalgia, and chronic pain syndromes.[26–28]

For these reasons, clinicians should be more cognizant of the possibility of PAD, particularly for patients with risk factors for this condition, and incorporate a pulse and skin assessment as a routine part of the examination for patients over the age of 40 years or those with the aforementioned risk factors. Findings such as pale white skin with elevation, erythema with limb lowering, areas of hair loss, poor wound healing, and in severe cases, distal ulceration can be seen. Palpation of peripheral pulses of the extremities usually reveals diminished or absent pulses distal to the site of stenosis. If one is unable to feel a pulse at a certain location, use of Doppler, if available, can be helpful to further assess the likelihood of PAD. A bruit may be heard at the interface between the stenotic lesion and upstream blood flow. Of note, the presence of either a diminished pulse or bruit significantly increases the likelihood of PAD.[29] **Fig. 1** provides an overview of the evaluation of a patient with suspected PAD.

A resting ankle-brachial index (ABI) should be performed on any patient, in which there is suspicion for PAD. In symptomatic individuals, a resting ABI of less than or equal to 0.90 is nearly 95% sensitive for detecting arteriogram-positive PAD and 100% specific in identifying healthy individuals.[30] Several studies have also correlated ABI cutoffs with symptom severity. These categories are as follows: ABI 0.9 to 0.4 is associated with intermittent claudication, ABI 0.4 to 0.2 is associated with rest pain, and ABI 0.4 to 0 is associated with gangrene/ulcers.[31–33] In addition, an ABI less than 0.90 correlated with a significant increased risk of 10-year cardiovascular mortality in both men and women with hazard ratios of 2.9 and 3.0, with adjustment for Framingham Risk Scoring.[34] Although the ABI has high diagnostic capability for detecting PAD, it is unable to reliably judge the severity or anatomical location of the vessel stenosis. Such patients should be referred to a vascular expert and additional imaging should be obtained such as duplex ultrasonography, computed tomography angiography (CTA), magnetic resonance angiography (MRA), or angiography. Of note, an ABI greater than 1.4 is also considered abnormal and usually indicates noncompressible vasculature, usually due to severe

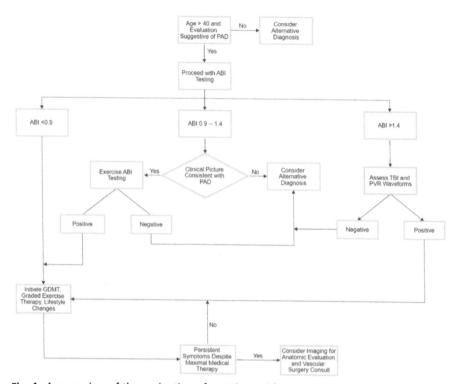

Fig. 1. An overview of the evaluation of a patient with suspected PAD. ABI, ankle brachial index; TBI, toe brachial index; PVR, pulse volume recording.

vessel calcification. Most common among those with diabetes, this finding should also be further investigated as ABIs greater than 1.4 correlate with major adverse cardiovascular events (MACEs).[35–37] A low toe-brachial index (TBI) is sometimes used in place of the ABI to diagnose PAD in patients with noncompressible vessels.[38,39]

For those patients who have symptoms suggestive of PAD, but a normal resting ABI, exercise testing is recommended. Although the American Heart Association (AHA) criteria for a postexercise ABI decrease of greater than 20% are widely used,[38] other methods including measuring transcutaneous PO_2 during exercise (with > 15 mm Hg delta of PO_2 being diagnostic of PAD) are also becoming widely accepted.[40–42] Using a combination of the above criteria including a postexercise ABI measurement (defined as a decrease of $\geq$ to 18.5%) and changes in the postexercise $TcPO_2$ demonstrated a significantly higher overall sensitivity.[43]

Key Points

- Fifty percent of patients with PAD are unaware of their disease, whereas 30% of providers do not know that their patients have PAD.
- Most of the patients with PAD either have atypical symptoms or are asymptomatic. Most patients with PAD *do not* present with classic, intermittent claudication.
- An ABI has excellent sensitivity and specificity for diagnosing PAD.
- An exercise ABI should be pursued in patients with a high suspicion for PAD who have a normal, resting ABI.

DISEASE CLASSIFICATION SCHEMES

Several classification schemes exist to stratify patients based on their initial disease burden. These systems are not intended to guide treatment decisions, but rather attempt to quantify disease burden and prognosis.

Both the Rutherford classification and Fontaine system have been widely used for decades. These classification schematics grade the severity of walking impairment using treadmill testing and a specific walking distance, respectively.[44,45] They also account for pain at rest as well as any tissue damage/loss associated with ischemic ulceration/gangrene. These classification systems were originally created to grade the severity of ischemia in patients with PAD alone but are becoming less reliable given the rising prevalence of diabetes, neuropathy, and other chronic illnesses that decrease the diagnostic usefulness of these systems through common symptomatology. The Wound, Ischemia, foot, Infection (WIfI) schematic, which uses a 0 to 3 scale to grade any wounds, severity of ischemia, and severity of foot infection if present, has become widely popular among vascular surgery societies as it is useful not only for initial staging of disease burden but also for restaging after intervention. The use of this scale has been validated by several studies demonstrating correlation with wound healing rate and time after 1 year.[46–48] It has also been helpful in determining the 1-year risk for major amputation rates.[49] Anatomical classification schemes also exist, such as the Trans-Atlantic Inter-Society Consensus, which defines arterial lesions as Type A, B, C, or D using anatomic distribution, number of lesions, types of lesions (stenosis, occlusions) and the predicted success rate of treatment using endovascular or surgical intervention. Such systems guide surgeons in treatment decisions, as short segments of vascular disease may be appropriately managed with endovascular intervention, while longer, more heavily occluded segments may require more aggressive surgical management.[30]

Key Points

- Several classification schemes exist to categorize PAD.
- The WIfI scheme is now endorsed by multiple societies to classify patients with limb-threatening ischemia.

MEDICAL THERAPY
Asymptomatic Disease

Patients with asymptomatic PAD represent a unique population that is poorly understood. Two large randomized clinical trials, the Prevention of Progression of Arterial Disease and Diabetes trial and the Aspirin for Asymptomatic Atherosclerosis trial, investigated the effect of aspirin on cardiovascular outcomes in patients with asymptomatic PAD.[50,51] Both trials found no significant difference in cardiovascular or cerebrovascular events between the aspirin and placebo groups. The American Heart Association/American College of Cardiology Guideline on the Management of Patients with Lower Extremity Peripheral Artery Disease from 2016 concluded that it is reasonable (grade IIa recommendation) to start antiplatelet therapy in patients with asymptomatic PAD if they have an ABI $\leq$ 0.9 to reduce the risk of major MACEs.[38] Because of a lack of proven benefit, the 2017 European Society of Cardiology Guideline on PAD did not recommend the routine use of antiplatelet therapy in patients with asymptomatic, isolated PAD.[52] The benefit of statin therapy in patients with asymptomatic PAD who lack other evidence of cardiovascular disease is also unclear. The American College of Cardiology suggests that statin therapy should be considered in all individuals with an atherosclerotic cardiovascular disease

(ASCVD) risk greater than 7.5%, which is commonly the case in all individuals with PAD.[53]

Key Points

- Randomized clinical trials did not show a cardiovascular benefit of antiplatelet therapy in asymptomatic PAD patients.
- The ACC guideline issued a grade IIa recommendation to start antiplatelet therapy in asymptomatic patients, given the lack of high-quality data supporting its use.
- It is reasonable to start statin therapy in patients with asymptomatic PAD, because most patients will likely have an ASVD risk score greater than 7.5%.

Symptomatic Disease

Antiplatelet/antithrombotic therapy

As platelet activation plays a fundamental role in atherosclerosis and arterial thrombosis, medical management of PAD includes antiplatelet and antithrombotic therapy.[38,54,55] The Antithrombotic Trialists' Collaboration conducted a meta-analysis of trials studying the efficacy of various antiplatelet agents in patients at high risk for occlusive vascular events, finding that antiplatelet therapy protects against vascular events in patients with stable angina, intermittent claudication, and atrial fibrillation.[56,57] Although the benefit of antiplatelet therapy for symptomatic PAD is undisputed, the choice of antiplatelet agent is debated. The Clopidogrel versus Aspirin in Patients at Risk of Ischemic Events (CAPRIE) trial demonstrated that daily clopidogrel reduced the risk of stroke and myocardial infarction (MI) more effectively when compared with aspirin in patients with a recent ischemic stroke, MI, or symptomatic PAD.[58] In fact, the PAD subgroup in this study experienced the greatest risk reduction with clopidogrel.[55,58] However, the use of even more potent antiplatelet monotherapy has not been consistently shown to incur additional benefit. Superiority for ticagrelor monotherapy, compared with clopidogrel, was not established in the EUCLID (Examining Use of Ticagrelor in Peripheral Artery Disease) trial.[59] The efficacy of dual-antiplatelet therapy was studied in the Clopidogrel for High Atherothrombotic Risk and Ischemic Stabilization, Management and Avoidance trial, which showed that the combination of clopidogrel and aspirin, compared with aspirin alone, had an overall neutral effect on most vascular outcomes but was associated an increased risk of bleeding complications.[60] Given the above studies, most guidelines recommend either aspirin or clopidogrel monotherapy in patients with symptomatic PAD.[38,52]

The combination of a vitamin k antagonist and antiplatelet therapy, compared with antiplatelet monotherapy, was associated with an increased risk of life-threatening bleeding without additional vascular benefit in the Warfarin Antiplatelet Vascular Evaluation trial.[61] However, more recent studies have analyzed the efficacy of dual-pathway inhibition (DPI), using a low dose of an anticoagulant in combination with antiplatelet therapy. Specifically, the Cardiovascular Outcomes for People Using Anticoagulation Strategies trial compared rivaroxaban (2.5 mg twice daily) plus aspirin to aspirin alone and rivaroxaban alone (5 mg twice daily) in patients with stable coronary and/or peripheral arterial disease. The rivaroxaban plus aspirin group had lower rates of cardiovascular death, stroke, or MI (MACEs) as well as major adverse limb events (MALEs) compared with the aspirin alone group, although with higher rates of bleeding.[62] DPI has also been studied in PAD patients who have undergone surgical management. Specifically, the VOYAGER (Vascular Outcomes Study of ASA [acetylsalicylic acid] Along with Rivaroxaban in Endovascular or Surgical Limb Revascularization) trial found that in patients with PAD who had undergone lower extremity revascularization, rivaroxaban added to daily aspirin reduced the risk of acute limb ischemia, MI, stroke, or cardiovascular death compared with aspirin alone.[63] The use of DPI therapy in daily clinical practice is evolving, and guideline recommendations regarding its use are forthcoming.

Key Points

- Aspirin or clopidogrel is recommended to lower the risk of MACEs in symptomatic PAD patients.
- Higher potency antiplatelet monotherapy (such as with ticagrelor) has not been consistently shown to provide additional cardiovascular benefit compared with lower potency antiplatelet monotherapy.
- Both high-dose anticoagulation and dual-antiplatelet therapy are associated with unfavorable risk/benefit profiles compared with antiplatelet monotherapy.
- DPI with low-dose rivaroxaban and aspirin lowers the risk of adverse cardiac and limb events, as compared with antiplatelet monotherapy, but is associated with a higher risk of bleeding. The risk/benefit profile for DPI likely becomes more favorable with higher baseline risks for cardiovascular events (such as those with polyvascular disease) or limb complications (such as those with prior episodes of limb-threatening ischemia or multiple revascularization procedures).

Lipid management

LDL-C plays a critical role in the development of atherosclerosis in peripheral arterial disease. The penetration of LDL into the arterial intima precipitates an inflammatory response involving reactive oxygen species, pro-inflammatory cytokines, and the recruitment of foamy macrophages and smooth muscle cells that ultimately leads to the formation of a plaque.[64] Reducing LDL lowers the risk of lower limb complications and the development of serious vascular events while halting the exacerbation of claudication symptoms.[52,64–67]

More recent data investigating the effects of inhibitors of proprotein convertase subtilisin–kexin type 9 (PCSK9) have shed additional light on the effects of LDL-C reductions in patients with atherosclerotic disease, including PAD patients. The Further Cardiovascular Outcomes Research with PCSK9 Inhibition in Subjects with Elevated Risk trial found that evolocumab, combined with statin therapy, lowered the risk of MACEs in patients with stable cardiovascular disease.[68] In this trial, 13.2% of all patients had established PAD. PAD patients treated with evolocumab had a significantly lower rate of MACE compared with patients only on statin therapy and the level of MACE reduction correlated with the degree of LDL lowering. In addition, all patients treated with evolocumab had a lower incidence of MALEs (acute limb ischemia, major amputation, or urgent revascularization).[69] Moreover, The Evaluation of Cardiovascular Outcomes After an Acute Coronary Syndrome During Treatment With Alirocumab trial demonstrated that the PCSK9 inhibitor, alirocumab, reduced the incidence of coronary death, MI, stroke, and unstable angina in patients with recent acute coronary syndrome and dyslipidemia compared with statin monotherapy.[70]

Given the above data, the European Atherosclerosis Society and European Society of Vascular Medicine guidelines recommend a goal LDL of less than 55 mg/dL in symptomatic PAD patients.[71] This LDL goal has also been most recently endorsed for patients with a very high risk of MACE (which includes most patients with symptomatic PAD) in the 2022 ACC Expert Consensus Decision Pathway for Integrating

Atherosclerotic Cardiovascular Disease and Multimorbidity Treatment statement. Typically, patients are started on statin therapy and the anti-lipid regimen is adjusted for the aforementioned LDL goal.[72] The role of lipoprotein(a) [Lp(a)] lowering in patients with cardiovascular disease is evolving. Studies have shown that elevated Lp(a) levels are an independent risk factor for PAD.[16,73] There are fewer studies analyzing the role of Lp(a) levels in secondary prevention of PAD complications after revascularization. Tomoi and colleagues found that in patients with PAD treated with revascularization, elevated Lp(a) levels were independently associated with MACE and MALE postsurgery, irrespective of LDL levels or statin use.[74] Although an elevated Lp(a) level is considered a risk-enhancing factor, guidelines have not established targeted Lp(a) levels, given a lack of high-quality evidence.

Key Points

- All patients with symptomatic PAD should be prescribed statin therapy, regardless of baseline LDL levels.
- The anti-lipid regimen should be adjusted to achieve a goal LDL of less than 55 mg/dL in most patients with symptomatic PAD.
- Although Lp(a) levels correlate with the risk of PAD and its complications, guidelines have not recommended interventions specifically targeting Lp(a).

Smoking cessation

Smoking cessation is critical in the treatment of PAD patients. The 2016 AHA/American College of Cardiology (ACC) Guideline on the Management of Patients with Lower Extremity Peripheral Artery Disease declared that patients with PAD who smoke tobacco should be advised at every visit to quit smoking. Physicians should assist patients in developing a plan for quitting that may involve referral to a smoking cessation program and/or pharmacotherapy such as varenicline, bupropion, and/or nicotine replacement therapy.[38]

Glycemic control

As stated earlier, diabetes is a known risk factor for PAD. The prevalence of PAD in patients with diabetes mellitus is estimated to be around 29%.[75] Furthermore, the atherosclerosis in diabetic patients with PAD is more aggressive, and amputation rates in diabetic patients with atherosclerosis of the lower extremity are much higher than non-diabetics.[76,77] The Society for Vascular Surgery suggests optimizing diabetes control (hemoglobin A1c goal of <7.0%) in patients with intermittent claudication.[76]

Blood pressure control

Hypertension is a known risk factor for PAD. The EUCLID trial found that in patients with symptomatic PAD, 78% had hypertension and that every 10 mm Hg increase in systolic blood pressure above 125 mm Hg was associated with an increased risk of MACE and an increased risk of MALE/lower extremity revascularization.[78] Similarly, multiple other trials have shown that blood pressure control is associated with improved cardiovascular outcomes in PAD patients.[79,80]

Sodium–glucose cotransporter-2 inhibitors and glucagon-like peptide-1 agonists

Both sodium–glucose cotransporter-2 (SGLT-2) inhibitors and glucagon-like peptide-1 (GLP-1) agonists are relatively new and promising antidiabetic drugs. The Empagliflozin Cardiovascular Outcome Event Trial in Type 2 Diabetes Mellitus Patients trial assessed cardiovascular outcomes in diabetic patients treated with empagliflozin and standard of care compared with placebo and standard of care. Empagliflozin significantly decreased the risk of cardiovascular disease (CVD) death, nonfatal MI, or nonfatal stroke compared with placebo.[81,82] Among patients with PAD, empagliflozin reduced all-cause and cardiovascular mortality, hospitalization for heart failure, and progression of renal disease.[81,83] The combined Canagliflozin Cardiovascular Assessment Study (CANVAS) and CANVAS-Renal trial studied patients with Type 2 diabetes mellitus (T2DM) on canagliflozin compared with placebo. Although canagliflozin reduced cardiovascular death, MI, and stroke rate, patients treated with canagliflozin were found to have a significantly higher rate of lower extremity amputation.[83,84] Interestingly, this increased amputation risk was not discovered in any other canagliflozin trial or trials with other SGLT-2 inhibitors. Yuan and colleagues conducted a retrospective review of patients with T2DM exposed to canagliflozin or non-SGLT2 antidiabetic agents and found that there was no increased risk of below-knee amputation in patients treated with canagliflozin.[83,85]

Data on the association and impact of GLP-1 agonists on PAD outcomes are more limited. Multiple retrospective reviews have found that in patients with T2DM, GLP-1 agonists were associated with a significant reduction in hospitalization for PAD and lower limb complications in comparison with other antidiabetic agents.[86-88] In addition, Marso and colleagues found that patients with T2DM treated with semaglutide had lower rates of peripheral revascularization than patients treated with placebo.[87,89]

Key Points

- Smoking cessation should be actively pursued in all patients with PAD.
- PAD patients with hypertension should be prescribed antihypertensive medications to achieve a goal blood pressure of less than 140/90. Both the American and European guidelines have issued grade IIa recommendations for angiotensin-converting enzyme inhibitors (ACEis) or angiotensin receptor blockers (ARBs) as initial therapy for hypertension in PAD patients.
- Data regarding the beneficial cardiovascular effects of SGLT-2 inhibitors and GLP-1 agonists specifically for PAD patients are emerging but promising.
- Early concerns regarding the amputation risk associated with certain SGLT-2 inhibitors have been allayed following analyses of recent data. The Food and Drug administration (FDA) has removed the black box warning of amputation for this class of drugs but advises prescribers to cautiously use this class of medications in patient at high risk of amputations, including PAD patients.

UNDERTREATMENT OF PERIPHERAL ARTERY DISEASE

When compared with CAD, there are substantially less clinical trials assessing the impact of medical management in regard to PAD.[90] However, it is still well-documented that statins and antiplatelet medications significantly reduce serious events associated with PAD.[38,91] Hess and colleagues conducted a review that showed that among roughly 250,000 PAD patients, 40% were not on any lipid-lowering therapy.[92] Furthermore, medical management was less likely to be used in black patient populations, with black women having the lowest rate of lipid-lowering therapy utilization.[93,94] Berger and Ladapo's study using the National Ambulatory Medical Care Survey and National Hospital Ambulatory Medical Care Survey databases ($n = 1982$) aimed at identifying outpatient physician trends in PAD management and found that only 38% of patients were on antiplatelet agents, 35% were on statins, and 31% used ACEi agents. In addition, exercise and diet were discussed only 20% of the time, and smoking cessation was addressed during 36% of encounters.[90] Even with the increased use of antiplatelet and statin therapy from 2006 to 2013, when demographics and comorbidities are controlled for, this increase is not significant.[90] Although the low rate of secondary prevention in the outpatient setting is not entirely understood, studies have demonstrated higher prescription rates in the hospital setting on discharge when compared with outpatient physician offices, a rather worrisome trend.[95–97] When compared with cardiologists, internists and family practitioners were significantly less likely to prescribe lipid lowering and antiplatelet agents, even though they see a substantially higher volume of PAD patients annually.[98]

One possible explanation may be the confounding findings of several antiplatelet trials. In the CAPRIE trial, clopidogrel was superior to aspirin in PAD patients compared with those with a history of stroke or CAD.[58] A subsequent meta-analysis found that aspirin is not as effective in preventing adverse cardiovascular outcomes in PAD as it is in CAD.[99] Given these findings, along with the recent EUCLID trial showing similar outcomes in PAD with Clopidogrel versus Ticagrelor,[59] there could be confusion regarding the appropriate medical management for patients with PAD who also have coexisting CAD.[100]

Key Points

- Historical and current data continue to highlight gaps of care for patients with PAD, compared with their CAD counterparts. The foundation of medical therapy for these patients, such as antiplatelet and statin therapy, is not used in the majority of cases.
- The undertreatment of PAD is even more profound in minority patients.

DISCLOSURE

T. Galanis, Consultant, Janssen Pharmaceuticals.

REFERENCES

1. Song P, Fang Z, Wang H, et al. Global and regional prevalence, burden, and risk factors for carotid atherosclerosis: a systematic review, meta-analysis, and modelling study. Lancet Glob Health 2020;8(5):e721–9.
2. Pande RL, Creager MA. Socioeconomic inequality and peripheral artery disease prevalence in US adults. Circ Cardiovasc Qual Outcomes 2014;7(4): 532–9.
3. Fowkes FG, Rudan D, Rudan I, et al. Comparison of global estimates of prevalence and risk factors for peripheral artery disease in 2000 and 2010: a systematic review and analysis. Lancet 2013;382(9901):1329–40.
4. Allison MA, Ho E, Denenberg JO, et al. Ethnic-specific prevalence of peripheral arterial disease in the United States. Am J Prev Med 2007;32(4):328–33.
5. Matsushita K, Sang Y, Ning H, et al. Lifetime Risk of Lower-Extremity Peripheral Artery Disease Defined by Ankle-Brachial Index in the United States. J Am Heart Assoc 2019;8(18):e012177.
6. Peripheral arterial disease in people with diabetes. Diabetes Care 2003;26(12): 3333–41.
7. Ding N, Sang Y, Chen J, et al. Cigarette Smoking, Smoking Cessation, and Long-Term Risk of 3 Major Atherosclerotic Diseases. J Am Coll Cardiol 2019; 74(4):498–507.
8. Khaleghi M, Isseh IN, Bailey KR, et al. Family history as a risk factor for peripheral arterial disease. Am J Cardiol 2014;114(6):928–32.

9. Lu Y, Ballew SH, Tanaka H, et al. 2017 ACC/AHA blood pressure classification and incident peripheral artery disease: The Atherosclerosis Risk in Communities (ARIC) Study. Eur J Prev Cardiol 2020;27(1):51–9.

10. Allison MA, Cushman M, Solomon C, et al. Ethnicity and risk factors for change in the ankle-brachial index: the Multi-Ethnic Study of Atherosclerosis. J Vasc Surg 2009;50(5):1049–56.

11. McDermott MM, Liu K, Criqui MH, et al. Ankle-brachial index and subclinical cardiac and carotid disease: the multi-ethnic study of atherosclerosis. Am J Epidemiol 2005;162(1):33–41.

12. Kennedy M, Solomon C, Manolio TA, et al. Risk factors for declining ankle-brachial index in men and women 65 years or older: the Cardiovascular Health Study. Arch Intern Med 2005;165(16):1896–902.

13. Ridker PM, Stampfer MJ, Rifai N. Novel risk factors for systemic atherosclerosis: a comparison of C-reactive protein, fibrinogen, homocysteine, lipoprotein(a), and standard cholesterol screening as predictors of peripheral arterial disease. JAMA 2001;285(19):2481–5.

14. Aday AW, Lawler PR, Cook NR, et al. Lipoprotein Particle Profiles, Standard Lipids, and Peripheral Artery Disease Incidence. Circulation 2018;138(21):2330–41.

15. Kou M, Ding N, Ballew SH, et al. Conventional and Novel Lipid Measures and Risk of Peripheral Artery Disease. Arterioscler Thromb Vasc Biol 2021;41(3):1229–38.

16. Tunstall-Pedoe H, Peters SAE, Woodward M, et al. Twenty-Year Predictors of Peripheral Arterial Disease Compared With Coronary Heart Disease in the Scottish Heart Health Extended Cohort (SHHEC). J Am Heart Assoc 2017;6(9). https://doi.org/10.1161/jaha.117.005967.

17. Arya S, Binney Z, Khakharia A, et al. Race and Socioeconomic Status Independently Affect Risk of Major Amputation in Peripheral Artery Disease. J Am Heart Assoc 2018;7(2). https://doi.org/10.1161/jaha.117.007425.

18. Fanaroff AC, Yang L, Nathan AS, et al. Geographic and Socioeconomic Disparities in Major Lower Extremity Amputation Rates in Metropolitan Areas. J Am Heart Assoc 2021;10(17):e021456.

19. Henry AJ, Hevelone ND, Belkin M, et al. Socioeconomic and hospital-related predictors of amputation for critical limb ischemia. J Vasc Surg 2011;53(2):330–9.e1.

20. Holman KH, Henke PK, Dimick JB, et al. Racial disparities in the use of revascularization before leg amputation in Medicare patients. J Vasc Surg 2011;54(2):420–6, 426.e1.

21. Selvarajah S, Black JH 3rd, Haider AH, et al. Racial disparity in early graft failure after infrainguinal bypass. J Surg Res 2014;190(1):335–43.

22. Eslami MH, Zayaruzny M, Fitzgerald GA. The adverse effects of race, insurance status, and low income on the rate of amputation in patients presenting with lower extremity ischemia. J Vasc Surg 2007;45(1):55–9.

23. Regenbogen SE, Gawande AA, Lipsitz SR, et al. Do differences in hospital and surgeon quality explain racial disparities in lower-extremity vascular amputations? Ann Surg 2009;250(3):424–31.

24. Novo S. Classification, epidemiology, risk factors, and natural history of peripheral arterial disease. Diabetes Obes Metab 2002;4(Suppl 2):S1–6.

25. Hirsch AT, Haskal ZJ, Hertzer NR, et al. ACC/AHA 2005 Practice Guidelines for the management of patients with peripheral arterial disease (lower extremity, renal, mesenteric, and abdominal aortic): a collaborative report from the

American Association for Vascular Surgery/Society for Vascular Surgery, Society for Cardiovascular Angiography and Interventions, Society for Vascular Medicine and Biology, Society of Interventional Radiology, and the ACC/AHA Task Force on Practice Guidelines (Writing Committee to Develop Guidelines for the Management of Patients With Peripheral Arterial Disease): endorsed by the American Association of Cardiovascular and Pulmonary Rehabilitation; National Heart, Lung, and Blood Institute; Society for Vascular Nursing; TransAtlantic Inter-Society Consensus; and Vascular Disease Foundation. Circulation 2006;113(11):e463–654.

26. Hirsch AT, Criqui MH, Treat-Jacobson D, et al. Peripheral arterial disease detection, awareness, and treatment in primary care. JAMA 2001;286(11):1317–24.

27. McDermott MM, Greenland P, Liu K, et al. Leg symptoms in peripheral arterial disease: associated clinical characteristics and functional impairment. JAMA 2001;286(13):1599–606.

28. Tendera M, Aboyans V, Bartelink ML, et al. ESC Guidelines on the diagnosis and treatment of peripheral artery diseases: Document covering atherosclerotic disease of extracranial carotid and vertebral, mesenteric, renal, upper and lower extremity arteries: the Task Force on the Diagnosis and Treatment of Peripheral Artery Diseases of the European Society of Cardiology (ESC). Eur Heart J 2011; 32(22):2851–906.

29. Khan NA, Rahim SA, Anand SS, et al. Does the clinical examination predict lower extremity peripheral arterial disease? JAMA 2006;295(5):536–46.

30. Norgren L, Hiatt WR, Dormandy JA, et al. Inter-Society Consensus for the Management of Peripheral Arterial Disease (TASC II). J Vasc Surg 2007;45(Suppl S): S5–67.

31. Mahé G, Le Faucheur A, Noury-Desvaux B. Ankle-brachial index and peripheral arterial disease. N Engl J Med 2010;362(5):470–1 [author reply: 471-2].

32. Parmenter BJ, Raymond J, Dinnen PJ, et al. Preliminary evidence that low ankle-brachial index is associated with reduced bilateral hip extensor strength and functional mobility in peripheral arterial disease. J Vasc Surg 2013;57(4): 963–73.e1.

33. Vierron E, Halimi JM, Giraudeau B. Ankle-brachial index and peripheral arterial disease. N Engl J Med 2010;362(5):471 [author reply: 471-2].

34. Fowkes FG, Murray GD, Butcher I, et al. Ankle brachial index combined with Framingham Risk Score to predict cardiovascular events and mortality: a meta-analysis. JAMA 2008;300(2):197–208.

35. McDermott MM, Applegate WB, Bonds DE, et al. Ankle brachial index values, leg symptoms, and functional performance among community-dwelling older men and women in the lifestyle interventions and independence for elders study. J Am Heart Assoc 2013;2(6):e000257.

36. Pasqualini L, Schillaci G, Pirro M, et al. Prognostic value of low and high ankle-brachial index in hospitalized medical patients. Eur J Intern Med 2012;23(3): 240–4.

37. Rac-Albu M, Iliuta L, Guberna SM, et al. The role of ankle-brachial index for predicting peripheral arterial disease. Maedica (Bucur) 2014;9(3):295–302.

38. Gerhard-Herman MD, Gornik HL, Barrett C, et al. 2016 AHA/ACC Guideline on the Management of Patients With Lower Extremity Peripheral Artery Disease: Executive Summary: A Report of the American College of Cardiology/American Heart Association Task Force on Clinical Practice Guidelines. J Am Coll Cardiol 2017;69(11):1465–508.

39. Halliday A, Bax JJ. The 2017 ESC Guidelines on the Diagnosis and Treatment of Peripheral Arterial Diseases, in Collaboration With the European Society for Vascular Surgery (ESVS). Eur J Vasc Endovasc Surg 2018;55(3):301–2.
40. Abraham P, Picquet J, Bouyé P, et al. Transcutaneous oxygen pressure measurements (tcpO2) at ankle during exercise in arterial claudication. Int Angiol 2005;24(1):80–8.
41. Abraham P, Picquet J, Vielle B, et al. Transcutaneous oxygen pressure measurements on the buttocks during exercise to detect proximal arterial ischemia: comparison with arteriography. Circulation 2003;107(14):1896–900.
42. Koch C, Chauve E, Chaudru S, et al. Exercise transcutaneous oxygen pressure measurement has good sensitivity and specificity to detect lower extremity arterial stenosis assessed by computed tomography angiography. Medicine (Baltim) 2016;95(36):e4522.
43. Stivalet O, Paisant A, Belabbas D, et al. Combination of Exercise Testing Criteria to Diagnose Lower Extremity Peripheral Artery Disease. Front Cardiovasc Med 2021;8:759666.
44. Rösler H. [Clinical significance of brain scintigraphy]. Fortschr Geb Rontgenstr Nuklearmed 1973;(suppl):67–8. Zur klinischen Wertigkeit der Hirnszintigraphie.
45. Rutherford RB, Baker JD, Ernst C, et al. Recommended standards for reports dealing with lower extremity ischemia: revised version. J Vasc Surg 1997; 26(3):517–38.
46. Darling JD, McCallum JC, Soden PA, et al. Predictive ability of the Society for Vascular Surgery Wound, Ischemia, and foot Infection (WIfI) classification system after first-time lower extremity revascularizations. J Vasc Surg 2017;65(3): 695–704.
47. Hicks CW, Canner JK, Karagozlu H, et al. The Society for Vascular Surgery Wound, Ischemia, and foot Infection (WIfI) classification system correlates with cost of care for diabetic foot ulcers treated in a multidisciplinary setting. J Vasc Surg 2018;67(5):1455–62.
48. Okazaki J, Matsuda D, Tanaka K, et al. Analysis of wound healing time and wound-free period as outcomes after surgical and endovascular revascularization for critical lower limb ischemia. J Vasc Surg 2018;67(3):817–25.
49. van Reijen NS, Ponchant K, Ubbink DT, et al. Editor's Choice - The Prognostic Value of the WIfI Classification in Patients with Chronic Limb Threatening Ischaemia: A Systematic Review and Meta-Analysis. Eur J Vasc Endovasc Surg 2019;58(3):362–71.
50. Belch J, MacCuish A, Campbell I, et al. The prevention of progression of arterial disease and diabetes (POPADAD) trial: factorial randomised placebo controlled trial of aspirin and antioxidants in patients with diabetes and asymptomatic peripheral arterial disease. BMJ 2008;337:a1840.
51. Fowkes FG, Price JF, Stewart MC, et al. Aspirin for prevention of cardiovascular events in a general population screened for a low ankle brachial index: a randomized controlled trial. JAMA 2010;303(9):841–8.
52. Aboyans V, Ricco JB, Bartelink MEL, et al. 2017 ESC Guidelines on the Diagnosis and Treatment of Peripheral Arterial Diseases, in collaboration with the European Society for Vascular Surgery (ESVS): Document covering atherosclerotic disease of extracranial carotid and vertebral, mesenteric, renal, upper and lower extremity arteriesEndorsed by: the European Stroke Organization (ESO)The Task Force for the Diagnosis and Treatment of Peripheral Arterial Diseases of the European Society of Cardiology (ESC) and of the European Society for Vascular Surgery (ESVS). Eur Heart J 2018;39(9):763–816.

53. Arnett DK, Blumenthal RS, Albert MA, et al. 2019 ACC/AHA Guideline on the Primary Prevention of Cardiovascular Disease: A Report of the American College of Cardiology/American Heart Association Task Force on Clinical Practice Guidelines. Circulation 2019;140(11):e596–646.

54. Alonso-Coello P, Bellmunt S, McGorrian C, et al. Antithrombotic therapy in peripheral artery disease: Antithrombotic Therapy and Prevention of Thrombosis, 9th ed: American College of Chest Physicians Evidence-Based Clinical Practice Guidelines. Chest 2012;141(2 Suppl):e669S–90S.

55. Hussain MA, Al-Omran M, Creager MA, et al. Antithrombotic Therapy for Peripheral Artery Disease: Recent Advances. J Am Coll Cardiol 2018;71(21):2450–67.

56. Collaborative overview of randomised trials of antiplatelet therapy–I: Prevention of death, myocardial infarction, and stroke by prolonged antiplatelet therapy in various categories of patients. Antiplatelet Trialists' Collaboration. BMJ 1994; 308(6921):81–106.

57. Collaborative meta-analysis of randomised trials of antiplatelet therapy for prevention of death, myocardial infarction, and stroke in high risk patients. Bmj 2002;324(7329):71–86.

58. A randomised, blinded, trial of clopidogrel versus aspirin in patients at risk of ischaemic events (CAPRIE). CAPRIE Steering Committee. Lancet 1996; 348(9038):1329–39.

59. Hiatt WR, Fowkes FG, Heizer G, et al. Ticagrelor versus Clopidogrel in Symptomatic Peripheral Artery Disease. N Engl J Med 2017;376(1):32–40.

60. Berger PB, Bhatt DL, Fuster V, et al. Bleeding complications with dual antiplatelet therapy among patients with stable vascular disease or risk factors for vascular disease: results from the Clopidogrel for High Atherothrombotic Risk and Ischemic Stabilization, Management, and Avoidance (CHARISMA) trial. Circulation 2010;121(23):2575–83.

61. Anand S, Yusuf S, Xie C, et al. Oral anticoagulant and antiplatelet therapy and peripheral arterial disease. N Engl J Med 2007;357(3):217–27.

62. Eikelboom JW, Connolly SJ, Bosch J, et al. Rivaroxaban with or without Aspirin in Stable Cardiovascular Disease. N Engl J Med 2017;377(14):1319–30.

63. Bonaca MP, Bauersachs RM, Anand SS, et al. Rivaroxaban in Peripheral Artery Disease after Revascularization. N Engl J Med 2020;382(21):1994–2004.

64. Jansen-Chaparro S, López-Carmona MD, Cobos-Palacios L, et al. Statins and Peripheral Arterial Disease: A Narrative Review. Front Cardiovasc Med 2021; 8:777016.

65. Randomized trial of the effects of cholesterol-lowering with simvastatin on peripheral vascular and other major vascular outcomes in 20,536 people with peripheral arterial disease and other high-risk conditions. J Vasc Surg 2007;45(4): 645–54 [discussion: 653-4].

66. Pedersen TR, Kjekshus J, Pyörälä K, et al. Effect of simvastatin on ischemic signs and symptoms in the Scandinavian simvastatin survival study (4S). Am J Cardiol 1998;81(3):333–5.

67. Stoekenbroek RM, Boekholdt SM, Fayyad R, et al. High-dose atorvastatin is superior to moderate-dose simvastatin in preventing peripheral arterial disease. Heart 2015;101(5):356–62.

68. Sabatine MS, Giugliano RP, Keech AC, et al. Evolocumab and Clinical Outcomes in Patients with Cardiovascular Disease. N Engl J Med 2017;376(18): 1713–22.

69. Wong ND, Shapiro MD. Interpreting the Findings From the Recent PCSK9 Monoclonal Antibody Cardiovascular Outcomes Trials. Front Cardiovasc Med 2019; 6:14.

70. Jukema JW, Szarek M, Zijlstra LE, et al. Alirocumab in Patients With Polyvascular Disease and Recent Acute Coronary Syndrome: ODYSSEY OUTCOMES Trial. J Am Coll Cardiol 2019;74(9):1167–76.

71. Belch JJF, Brodmann M, Baumgartner I, et al. Lipid-lowering and antithrombotic therapy in patients with peripheral arterial disease: European Atherosclerosis Society/European Society of Vascular Medicine Joint Statement. Atherosclerosis 2021;338:55–63.

72. Birtcher KK, Allen LA, Anderson JL, et al. 2022 ACC Expert Consensus Decision Pathway for Integrating Atherosclerotic Cardiovascular Disease and Multimorbidity Treatment: A Framework for Pragmatic, Patient-Centered Care: A Report of the American College of Cardiology Solution Set Oversight Committee. J Am Coll Cardiol 2023;81(3):292–317.

73. Gurdasani D, Sjouke B, Tsimikas S, et al. Lipoprotein(a) and risk of coronary, cerebrovascular, and peripheral artery disease: the EPIC-Norfolk prospective population study. Arterioscler Thromb Vasc Biol 2012;32(12):3058–65.

74. Tomoi Y, Takahara M, Soga Y, et al. Impact of High Lipoprotein(a) Levels on Clinical Outcomes Following Peripheral Endovascular Therapy. JACC Cardiovasc Interv 2022;15(14):1466–76.

75. Elhadd TA, Jung RT, Newton RW, et al. Incidence of asymptomatic peripheral arterial occlusive disease in diabetic patients attending a hospital clinic. Adv Exp Med Biol 1997;428:45–8.

76. Conte MS, Pomposelli FB, Clair DG, et al. Society for Vascular Surgery practice guidelines for atherosclerotic occlusive disease of the lower extremities: management of asymptomatic disease and claudication. J Vasc Surg 2015;61(3 Suppl):2s–41s.

77. Soyoye DO, Abiodun OO, Ikem RT, et al. Diabetes and peripheral artery disease: A review. World J Diabetes 2021;12(6):827–38.

78. Fudim M, Hopley CW, Huang Z, et al. Association of Hypertension and Arterial Blood Pressure on Limb and Cardiovascular Outcomes in Symptomatic Peripheral Artery Disease: The EUCLID Trial. Circ Cardiovasc Qual Outcomes 2020; 13(9):e006512.

79. Bavry AA, Anderson RD, Gong Y, et al. Outcomes Among hypertensive patients with concomitant peripheral and coronary artery disease: findings from the INternational VErapamil-SR/Trandolapril STudy. Hypertension 2010;55(1):48–53.

80. Yusuf S, Sleight P, Pogue J, et al. Effects of an angiotensin-converting-enzyme inhibitor, ramipril, on cardiovascular events in high-risk patients. N Engl J Med 2000;342(3):145–53.

81. Verma S, Mazer CD, Al-Omran M, et al. Cardiovascular Outcomes and Safety of Empagliflozin in Patients With Type 2 Diabetes Mellitus and Peripheral Artery Disease: A Subanalysis of EMPA-REG OUTCOME. Circulation 2018;137(4): 405–7.

82. Zinman B, Wanner C, Lachin JM, et al. Empagliflozin, Cardiovascular Outcomes, and Mortality in Type 2 Diabetes. N Engl J Med 2015;373(22):2117–28.

83. Chatterjee S, Bandyopadhyay D, Ghosh RK, et al. SGLT-2 Inhibitors and Peripheral Artery Disease: A Statistical Hoax or Reality? Curr Probl Cardiol 2019;44(7): 207–22.

84. Neal B, Perkovic V, Mahaffey KW, et al. Canagliflozin and Cardiovascular and Renal Events in Type 2 Diabetes. N Engl J Med 2017;377(7):644–57.

85. Yuan Z, DeFalco FJ, Ryan PB, et al. Risk of lower extremity amputations in people with type 2 diabetes mellitus treated with sodium-glucose co-transporter-2 inhibitors in the USA: A retrospective cohort study. Diabetes Obes Metab 2018;20(3):582–9.

86. Baviera M, Genovese S, Lepore V, et al. Lower risk of death and cardiovascular events in patients with diabetes initiating glucagon-like peptide-1 receptor agonists or sodium-glucose cotransporter-2 inhibitors: A real-world study in two Italian cohorts. Diabetes Obes Metab 2021;23(7):1484–95.

87. Liarakos AL, Tentolouris A, Kokkinos A, et al. Impact of Glucagon-like peptide 1 receptor agonists on peripheral arterial disease in people with diabetes mellitus: A narrative review. J Diabetes Complications 2023;37(2):108390.

88. O'Brien MJ, Karam SL, Wallia A, et al. Association of Second-line Antidiabetic Medications With Cardiovascular Events Among Insured Adults With Type 2 Diabetes. JAMA Netw Open 2018;1(8):e186125.

89. Marso SP, Bain SC, Consoli A, et al. Semaglutide and Cardiovascular Outcomes in Patients with Type 2 Diabetes. N Engl J Med 2016;375(19):1834–44.

90. Berger JS, Ladapo JA. Underuse of Prevention and Lifestyle Counseling in Patients With Peripheral Artery Disease. J Am Coll Cardiol 2017;69(18):2293–300.

91. Berger JS, Hiatt WR. Medical therapy in peripheral artery disease. Circulation 2012;126(4):491–500.

92. Hess CN, Cannon CP, Beckman JA, et al. Effectiveness of Blood Lipid Management in Patients With Peripheral Artery Disease. J Am Coll Cardiol 2021;77(24): 3016–27.

93. Amrock SM, Duell PB, Knickelbine T, et al. Health disparities among adult patients with a phenotypic diagnosis of familial hypercholesterolemia in the CASCADE-FH™ patient registry. Atherosclerosis 2017;267:19–26.

94. Nanna MG, Navar AM, Zakroysky P, et al. Association of Patient Perceptions of Cardiovascular Risk and Beliefs on Statin Drugs With Racial Differences in Statin Use: Insights From the Patient and Provider Assessment of Lipid Management Registry. JAMA Cardiol 2018;3(8):739–48.

95. Armstrong EJ, Chen DC, Westin GG, et al. Adherence to guideline-recommended therapy is associated with decreased major adverse cardiovascular events and major adverse limb events among patients with peripheral arterial disease. J Am Heart Assoc 2014;3(2):e000697.

96. Cacoub PP, Abola MT, Baumgartner I, et al. Cardiovascular risk factor control and outcomes in peripheral artery disease patients in the Reduction of Atherothrombosis for Continued Health (REACH) Registry. Atherosclerosis 2009; 204(2):e86–92.

97. Subherwal S, Patel MR, Kober L, et al. Missed opportunities: despite improvement in use of cardioprotective medications among patients with lower-extremity peripheral artery disease, underuse remains. Circulation 2012; 126(11):1345–54.

98. McDermott MM, Hahn EA, Greenland P, et al. Atherosclerotic risk factor reduction in peripheral arterial diseasea: results of a national physician survey. J Gen Intern Med 2002;17(12):895–904.

99. Berger JS, Lala A, Krantz MJ, et al. Aspirin for the prevention of cardiovascular events in patients without clinical cardiovascular disease: a meta-analysis of randomized trials. Am Heart J 2011;162(1):115–24.e2.

100. Hiatt WR, Rogers RK. The Treatment Gap in Peripheral Artery Disease. J Am Coll Cardiol 2017;69(18):2301–3.

Peripheral Artery Disease
Treatment of Claudication and Surgical Management

Matthew Bierowski, MD[a], Taki Galanis, MD[b],*,
Amry Majeed, MD[a], Alireza Mofid, MD[c]

KEYWORDS

- Peripheral artery disease • Claudication • Ankle-brachial index • Limb ischemia

KEY POINTS

- Peripheral artery disease (PAD) is common and affects approximately 230 and 5 million people worldwide and nationally, respectively.
- Race and socioeconomic status have profound impacts on PAD outcomes.
- PAD is an under-recognized and under-treated medical condition.

TREATMENT OF CLAUDICATION

Therapy for claudication is aimed at improving functional capacity and quality of life. Pharmacologic therapies, such as pentoxifylline and cilastazol, for peripheral artery disease (PAD) have produced inconsistent results and are not endorsed by guidelines as the standard of care.[1,2] Therefore, aerobic exercise therapy (ET) and lower extremity revascularization (LER) are the preferred management strategies.[1,3,4] Biswas and colleagues found that aerobic ET and LER both improved peak walking performance and quality of life over non-intervention. Most guidelines recommend an exercise-only approach as initial management for claudication. However, if this is unsuccessful, the combination of ET and LER is likely superior to either intervention alone.[1]

The two main modalities for aerobic ET are supervised exercise therapy (SET) and home-based exercise therapy (HBET). SET, which has been approved by Medicare, involves a formal program with the majority of exercises involving walking or training lower extremities most often under the supervision of a physical therapist. HBET involves walking advice given by a clinician in addition to exercise monitoring through

---

[a] Internal Medicine, Thomas Jefferson University Hospital, 1025 Walnut Street, Philadelphia, PA 19107, USA; [b] Division Vascular Medicine, Jefferson Vascular Center, Sidney Kimmel Medical College, Philadelphia, PA, USA; [c] Vascular Surgery, Thomas Jefferson University Hospital, 111 South 11th Street, Suite 6210 Gibbon, Philadelphia, PA 19107, USA
* Corresponding author. 111 South 11th Street, Suite 6210 Gibbon, Philadelphia, PA 19107.
E-mail address: Taki.Galanis@jefferson.edu

Med Clin N Am 107 (2023) 823–827
https://doi.org/10.1016/j.mcna.2023.05.008
0025-7125/23/© 2023 Elsevier Inc. All rights reserved.

logbooks or pedometers.[5,6] SET has been shown to be superior to HBET for treadmill-measured walking distance. However, in many cases, HBET is preferred due to advantages in cost and convenience.[6,7] The Low-Intensity Exercise Intervention in PAD trial showed that a high-intensity, home-based exercise regimen, which involves exercising to induce ischemic symptoms, was superior to low-intensity exercise in improving walking distances in patients with PAD.[8] Overall, studies have found that HBET may be superior to ET for quality of life measures. However, most successful HBET trials involved intensive intervention (frequent training and feedback sessions, support groups, etc.) that may be difficult to replicate in real-world settings.

Key Points

- Exercise therapy is the first-line treatment of claudication and is a Medicare-approved intervention.
- The choice of supervised exercise therapy (SET) versus home-based exercise therapy (HBET) will depend on patient preferences and local resources. If a decision is made to pursue HBET, it must remain structured and intense.
- Re-vascularization is often reserved for those patients who fail medical therapy or have profound symptoms at baseline.

SURGICAL INTERVENTION
Indications for Intervention

There are two major indications for surgical or endovascular revascularization of patients with PAD. The first indication is lifestyle-limiting claudication to the extent where claudication is severely impacting a patient's quality of life or daily occupation. The second major indication involves critical limb ischemia (CLI) characterized by rest pain, tissue loss, or both. The main goal of treatment in patients with CLI is to reduce ischemic pain, improve limb preservation, and enhance amputation-free survival.[9,10]

Preoperative assessment

The preoperative assessment of patients undergoing revascularization begins with a thorough history and physical examination followed by targeted imaging investigations to evaluate the extent and level of PAD. It is important to identify a history of co-morbidities such as major cardiopulmonary disease, as presence of concurrent comorbidities can impact decision-making regarding endovascular therapy versus open surgical revascularization. Patients in whom open surgery is too risky will be offered endovascular revascularization. As such, a complete cardiopulmonary risk assessment is an important part of the pre-operative evaluation.[11]

It is also important to determine the extent of ischemic extremity pain and tissue loss. It is imperative to tease out the distance a patient can walk before claudication occurs and whether claudication is affecting the patient's day-to-day life. For the majority of patients, revascularization may be offered when a patient is unable to walk more than one city block before needing to stop to achieve relief of claudication, despite maximal medical therapy. There is a subset of patients, however, who will be offered revascularization at a longer distance of claudication onset due to severe limitation of their lifestyle and occupation. A classic example of this would be a postal service worker who is unable to perform his/her daily occupational tasks due to the onset of claudication at five blocks despite maximal medical therapy. In this scenario, a more aggressive revascularization plan should be offered to improve the patient's quality of life.[9,12] With regards to targeted imaging of patients with PAD, the first step is to obtain an ankle-brachial index (ABI), a non-invasive ultrasound-based modality that can provide substantial information on the status of peripheral circulation.

Other imaging modalities that can provide additional information regarding the location and degree of stenosis are duplex ultrasound and computed tomographic arteriogram of the abdomen and pelvis with run-off.[9]

Once patients with suspected PAD are referred to a vascular surgeon, they may undergo a peripheral angiogram, which is an invasive modality and the gold standard for diagnosing PAD. Angiography provides real-time imaging of contrast flow within the arterial system and can simultaneously provide valuable information on severity of PAD and be therapeutic for patients whose disease is amenable to endovascular therapy.[9]

Endovascular therapy vs. open surgery
The decision algorithm to treat PAD patients with endovascular therapy over open surgery is complex and multifactorial. Typically, healthier and younger patients are offered open surgery as the initial treatment due to superior durability of open surgery compared with endovascular therapy. If a patient is physiologically intolerant of open surgery, endovascular treatment is often pursued. However, a critical requirement in these patients is whether the lesion of interest is anatomically amenable to endovascular therapy. The Trans-Atlantic Inter-Society Consensus Document on Management of Peripheral Arterial Disease (TASC II) has put forward general guidelines with regard to which lesions should ideally be treated with open surgery versus endovascular treatment. In short, the TASC guidelines recommend endovascular balloon angioplasty and/or stenting for focal, short segment stenoses, whereas longer stenoses and arterial occlusions should ideally be treated with open surgery, if possible.[9]

Post-operative surveillance
Following endovascular treatment, patients are often prescribed dual-antiplatelet therapy (DAPT). Data on the optimal length of DAPT vary and are often provider-dependent. Typically, patients remain on DAPT for 1 to 6 months followed by indefinite antiplatelet monotherapy. Patients who have undergone open infra-inguinal bypass surgery are prescribed indefinite antiplatelet monotherapy, as this has been shown to significantly reduce the risk of bypass thrombosis.[13,14]

The Society of Vascular Surgery (SVS) has published general guidelines on the surveillance of patients who have undergone treatment of peripheral vascular disease. SVS guidelines recommend early post-operative follow-up for open bypass patients with a baseline ABI and clinical examination, which is then repeated at the 6 and 12 month intervals and yearly thereafter. The follow-up intervals are shortened if the patient develops recurrence of symptoms. This follow-up regimen can be with or without the addition of duplex ultrasound. In patients who have undergone endovascular therapy for PAD, the SVS guidelines recommend clinical examination, ABI, and duplex ultrasound within the first post-operative month. After the first month, guidelines differ based on the anatomic level of revascularization. Patients who have undergone treatment of aorto-iliac disease are followed at 6 and 12 months with clinical examination and ABI, and then yearly if there are no new symptoms. The SVS guidelines recommend continued surveillance of patients who have undergone endovascular treatment of femoropopliteal and tibial disease at 3 months and then every 6 months, though the strength of this recommendation is low. Owing to lack of consensus regarding surveillance of patients after endovascular treatment, in a real-world clinical setting, these patients are often evaluated at 1, 6, and 12 months, then annually thereafter.[15,16]

During post-operative surveillance, a decrease in the ABI of greater than 0.15 suggests potential disease recurrence and should prompt further investigation with duplex ultrasonography to confirm and identify the location of stenosis. On duplex ultrasound, one can observe low flow volumes at the site of stenosis with increased peak systolic velocity, and an increase in the velocity ratio between the site of investigation compared with the vessel proximal to the site of stenosis. In symptomatic patients, the presence of anastomotic stenosis due to neointimal hyperplasia in bypass grafts or within stents causing in-stent restenosis is an indication for potential intervention with a drug-eluted balloon angioplasty. Drug-eluted balloons are coated with pacli-taxel, an antiproliferative agent, shown which has been shown to reduce neointimal hyperplasia. Drug-eluted balloons have demonstrated superior outcomes compared with plain balloons with regard to treatment and prevention of re-stenosis.[15,17–20]

Key Points

- Surgical intervention is generally reserved for persistent symptoms that interfere with a patient's quality of life, despite exercise therapy or in those with profound baseline discomfort and/or limb-threatening ischemia.
- The choice of intervention (open versus endovascular) will depend on the patient's co-morbidities and extent of disease burden.
- Post-operative surveillance often involves at least a clinical and ABI assessment at pre-defined intervals. Changes in the clinical status of a patient (ie, new-onset or worsening pain), an ABI decrease of greater than 0.15, high velocity ratios, or very low absolute velocities in bypass grafts, warrant an immediate assessment by a vascular specialist.

DISCLOSURE

T. Galanis, Consultant, Janssen Pharmaceuticals.

REFERENCES

1. Biswas MP, Capell WH, McDermott MM, et al. Exercise training and revascularization in the management of symptomatic peripheral artery disease. JACC Basic Transl Sci 2021;6(2):174–88.
2. Hiatt WR. Treatment of disability in peripheral arterial disease: new drugs. Curr Drug Targets Cardiovasc Haematol Disord 2004;4(3):227–31.
3. Aboyans V, Ricco JB, Bartelink MEL, et al. 2017 ESC Guidelines on the Diagnosis and Treatment of Peripheral Arterial Diseases, in collaboration with the European Society for Vascular Surgery (ESVS): Document covering atherosclerotic disease of extracranial carotid and vertebral, mesenteric, renal, upper and lower extremity arteriesEndorsed by: the European Stroke Organization (ESO)The Task Force for the Diagnosis and Treatment of Peripheral Arterial Diseases of the European Society of Cardiology (ESC) and of the European Society for Vascular Surgery (ESVS). Eur Heart J 2018;39(9):763–816.
4. Gerhard-Herman MD, Gornik HL, Barrett C, et al. 2016 AHA/ACC guideline on the management of patients with lower extremity peripheral artery disease: executive summary: a report of the American college of cardiology/American heart association task force on clinical practice guidelines. J Am Coll Cardiol 2017;69(11): 1465–508.
5. Hageman D, Fokkenrood HJ, Gommans LN, et al. Supervised exercise therapy versus home-based exercise therapy versus walking advice for intermittent claudication. Cochrane Database Syst Rev 2018;4(4):Cd005263.
6. McDermott MM, Polonsky TS. Home-based exercise: a therapeutic option for peripheral artery disease. Circulation 2016;134(16):1127–9.

7. Harwood AE, Smith GE, Cayton T, et al. A systematic review of the uptake and adherence rates to supervised exercise programs in patients with intermittent claudication. Ann Vasc Surg 2016;34:280–9.
8. McDermott MM, Spring B, Tian L, et al. Effect of low-intensity vs high-intensity home-based walking exercise on walk distance in patients with peripheral artery disease: the LITE randomized clinical trial. JAMA 2021;325(13):1266–76.
9. Norgren L, Hiatt WR, Dormandy JA, et al. Inter-society consensus for the management of peripheral arterial disease (TASC II). J Vasc Surg 2007;45(Suppl S):S5–67.
10. Vartanian SM, Conte MS. Surgical intervention for peripheral arterial disease. Circ Res 2015;116(9):1614–28.
11. Durrand JW, Danjoux GR. Preoperative assessment of patients for major vascular surgery. Anaesth Intensive Care Med 2022;23(4):197–201.
12. Imparato AM, Kim GE, Davidson T, et al. Intermittent claudication: its natural course. Surgery 1975;78(6):795–9.
13. Aday AW, Gutierrez JA. Antiplatelet therapy following peripheral arterial interventions: the choice is yours. Circ Cardiovasc Interv 2020;13(8):e009727.
14. Yang JK, Jimenez JC, Jabori S. Antiplatelet therapy before, during, and after extremity revascularization. J Vasc Surg 2014;60(4):1085–91.
15. Sobieszczyk P, Eisenhauer A. Management of patients after endovascular interventions for peripheral artery disease. Circulation 2013;128(7):749–57.
16. Zierler RE, Jordan WD, Lal BK, et al. The society for vascular surgery practice guidelines on follow-up after vascular surgery arterial procedures. J Vasc Surg 2018;68(1):256–84.
17. Aboyans V, Criqui MH, Abraham P, et al. Measurement and interpretation of the ankle-brachial index: a scientific statement from the American Heart Association. Circulation 2012;126(24):2890–909.
18. Cassese S, Wolf F, Ingwersen M, et al. Drug-coated balloon angioplasty for femoropopliteal in-stent restenosis. Circ Cardiovasc Interv 2018;11(12):e007055.
19. Hodgkiss-Harlow KD, Bandyk DF. Interpretation of arterial duplex testing of lower-extremity arteries and interventions. Semin Vasc Surg 2013;26(2–3):95–104.
20. Promoting an increased awareness and standardized approaches in diagnosing and treating peripheral artery disease. The Society for Vascular Medicine. Available at: https://myperipheralarterydisease.com/health-care-providers/algorithmic-approach-and-pathway-to-pad-diagnosis/arterial-duplex-ultrasonography/.

Cold Hands or Feet
Is It Raynaud's or Not?

Daniella Kadian-Dodov, MD

KEYWORDS

- Raynaud's phenomenon • Raynaud's disease • Vasospasm
- Cold-induced vasospasm • Raynaud

KEY POINTS

- Raynaud's phenomenon is an exaggerated response to cold stimuli that may be primary or secondary in etiology.
- Raynaud's phenomenon refers to cold-induced vasospasm resulting in at least two phases of color change: pallor and cyanosis/rubor.
- Primary Raynaud's phenomenon (Raynaud disease) is defined by (1) intermittent attacks with complete resolution, (2) bilateral findings, (3) absence of organic occlusion, (4) changes limited to the superficial skin, and (5) symptoms for at least 2 years with no other explanation.

INTRODUCTION

Maurice Raynaud first described "local asphyxia and symmetric extremity gangrene" in 1862.[1] Classically, Raynaud's phenomenon (RP) is described as transient and exaggerated discoloration of the hands and/or feet with cold or stress exposures.[2,3] Up to three phases are described, although patients may not experience all phases (**Fig. 1**): first, pallor due to digital artery vasospasm and ischemia; second, cyanosis due to postcapillary venule constriction and deoxygenation of stagnant blood; third, rubor due to vasodilation and reactive hyperemia.[2,4,5] Raynaud's phenomenon may be primary (PRP) or secondary (SRP) due to underlying conditions, such as rheumatologic disease, vaso-occlusive disease, hematologic disorders, anatomic causes, infection, or environmental and drug exposure (**Table 1**). PRP is a diagnosis of exclusion with specific criteria (**Table 2**).[6] There are a number of conditions resulting in vasomotor dysfunction that the provider must consider when evaluating a patient with cold hands and feet, including acrocyanosis, pernio, small fiber neuropathy (SFN) with vasomotor symptoms, and complex regional pain syndrome (CRPS). This article outlines the diagnostic and treatment approach to the patient presenting with symptoms of suspected RP.

Zena and Michael A. Wiener Cardiovascular Institute, Icahn School of Medicine at Mount Sinai, 1190 Fifth Avenue, Box 1030, New York, NY 10029, USA
E-mail address: daniella.kadian-dodov@mountsinai.org

Med Clin N Am 107 (2023) 829–844
https://doi.org/10.1016/j.mcna.2023.04.005
0025-7125/23/© 2023 Elsevier Inc. All rights reserved.

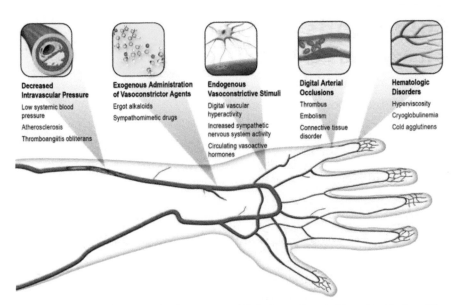

Decreased Intravascular Pressure
Low systemic blood pressure
Atherosclerosis
Thromboangiitis obliterans

Exogenous Administration of Vasoconstrictor Agents
Ergot alkaloids
Sympathomimetic drugs

Endogenous Vasoconstrictive Stimuli
Digital vascular hyperactivity
Increased sympathetic nervous system activity
Circulating vasoactive hormones

Digital Arterial Occlusions
Thrombus
Embolism
Connective tissue disorder

Hematologic Disorders
Hyperviscosity
Cryoglobulinemia
Cold agglutinens

Fig. 1. Mechanisms of Raynaud's phenomenon (digital vasospasm). (*From* Henkin S and Creager MA. Raynaud's Phenomenon. In: Creager MA, Beckman JA, Loscalzo J, eds. Vascular Medicine: A Companion to Braunwald's Heart Disease. 3ed. Philadelphia: Elsevier; 2020: 625-639.)

NATURE OF THE PROBLEM

RP is a common problem that affects women more than men. The true prevalence and incidence of RP are difficult to ascertain due to a lack of uniformity in definition. Most surveys and consensus panels agree that digital pallor triggered by cold exposure is needed for the diagnosis of RP and that the patient should experience at least two of the possible three phases of discoloration.[5,7–12] Some patients may additionally experience RP with emotional triggers. The pathophysiology of RP is thought to be a conglomeration of factors leading to exaggerated digital vasospasm resulting in transient ischemia (**Fig. 2**).[3,13]

The reported prevalence is 12% to 15% of patients in Northern European ambulatory populations.[8–10] Slightly lower rates (11% women, 8% men) are reported in US community-based studies, although a predilection for female sex persists across location.[11] Annual rates of RP incidence are higher in northern latitudes (0.7% in women and 0.9% in men from Northern Sweden) compared with more southern latitudes (0.3% in women and 0.2% in men in Northeast United States).[8,11] The mean age of diagnosis is around 34 years with a delay from symptom onset to diagnosis of 3 to 4 years.[8,12]

Most of the patients will have PRP, which has been associated with female sex, family history, and migraine headaches.[14,15] Over time, about one-third of patients will experience persistent RP and two-thirds will have remittance of disease.[11] By definition, PRP does not result in tissue loss or gangrene, although symptoms can be disconcerting and uncomfortable for the affected patient.[6]

Secondary causes of RP are identified in roughly 5% of patients, and most often due to autoimmune connective tissue diseases. Over time, reversible vasospasm may lead to fixed small vessel obstruction and digital ischemia—this is a particularly important distinction for the application of diagnostic testing as noted below.

Table 1
Causes of Raynaud's phenomenon

Primary Raynaud's Phenomenon (Raynaud's Disease)	Female sex Migraine headaches Family history of PRP
Secondary Raynaud's phenomenon	
Rheumatologic disease	Systemic and limited sclerosis Sjogren's syndrome Mixed connective tissue disease Dermatomyositis/polymyositis Systemic lupus erythematosus Antiphospholipid antibody syndrome
Vaso-occlusive disease	Atherosclerosis Thromboembolic Thromboangiitis obliterans
Hematologic disorders	Paraproteinemia Cryoglobulins Cold agglutinins Polycythemia POEMS (polyneuropathy, organomegaly, endocrinopathy, monoclonal protein skin changes) Cryofibrinogenemia
Drug-induced[24]	Ergots Amphetamines Sympathomimetics Poly vinyl chloride Chemotherapeutic agents
Environmental	Vibratory injury Trauma (eg, hypothenar hammer syndrome) Frostbite
Infection related	Hepatitis B or C (cryoglobulins) Mycoplasma (cold agglutinins)
Anatomic	Thoracic outlet syndrome Carpal tunnel syndrome

EVALUATION AND DIAGNOSIS

The evaluation of suspected RP begins with a thorough history and physical examination to identify distinguishing features in the differential diagnosis (see **Table 2**). RP classically presents with discoloration that is completely reversible, in contrast to acrocyanosis which results in constant discoloration that may wax and wane in severity.[16] The presence of skin ulceration or ischemia excludes the possibility of PRP.[6] Cold-induced vasospasm resulting in itching, swelling, or burning of the distal digits is characteristic of pernio and can occur concomitantly with RP or acrocyanosis.[17,18] A history of recent COVID-19 infection may also point to pernio in this setting.[19] Achenbach syndrome occurs suddenly as blue discoloration of a digit but is typically constant in discoloration, may be painful, and resolves with resolution of the spontaneous venous hemorrhage.[20] SFN with vasomotor symptoms or CRPS may be difficult to differentiate, although typically exhibit discoloration independent of cold exposure and may have accompanying symptoms of temperature intolerance, swelling, numbness, or tingling that are not typically seen in RP.[21,22] History of nerve injury may additionally help to clarify the diagnosis of CRPS.

Table 2
Differential diagnosis of Raynaud's phenomenon

	Criteria or Distinguishing Features	Mechanism of Skin Findings
Raynaud's disease (Primary Raynaud's phenomenon)[6]	1. Intermittent attacks 2. Absence of organic occlusion 3. Bilateral findings 4. Changes limited to superficial skin (no ulcers) 5. Absence of systemic disease to account for symptoms 6. Symptoms present for at least 2 y	Completely reversible vasospasm of the digital arteries resulting in discoloration with no fixed obstruction
Secondary Raynaud's phenomenon	1. Intermittent attacks 2. Skin findings (eg pitting), ulcerations, gangrene can occur 3. Abnormal physiologic testing or nailfold capillaroscopy 4. Clinical course is related to underlying etiology	Vasospasm of the digital arteries resulting in discoloration that may be in response to, or lead to, fixed obstruction of the small arteries
Pernio "Chilblains"[17,19]	1. Macules, papules, or patches of red, purple, or yellow discoloration on the digital pads or surrounding the nail beds 2. Symptom onset in colder months with resolution in warmer weather that may include swelling, numbness, itching, and burning of the digits 3. May ulcerate with repeated exposure, but does not cause gangrene 4. Rarely, secondary to COVID-19 or inflammatory disease such as lupus.	Reversible cold-induced small vessel vasospasm leading to an inflammatory reaction in the tissue. Can coexist with RP and acrocyanosis.
Acrocyanosis[16]	1. Constant blue discoloration with periodic worsening (color never fully normalizes) 2. Discoloration may extend up to the ankle/wrist 3. Color normalizes when the limb is raised above the level of the heart 4. Non-painful 5. Hyperhidrosis (ie, clammy skin) is common	Cutaneous vasoconstriction with capillary and subcapillary venous plexus dilation

Complex regional pain syndrome[21]	1. Continuing pain disproportionate to any inciting event	Multifaceted syndrome involving both central and peripheral pathophysiology. May have history of nerve injury.
	2. Must report one symptom in *three of the four* following categories:	
	a. Sensory: hyperalgesia, allodynia	
	b. Vasomotor: temperature asymmetry and/or skin color changes and/or skin color asymmetry	
	c. Sudomotor/edema: edema and/or sweating changes and/or sweating asymmetry	
	d. Motor/trophic: decreased range of motion and/or motor dysfunction (weakness, tremor, dystonia) and/or trophic changes (hair, nail, skin)	
	3. Must display at least one sign at the time of evaluation in *two or more* of the following categories:	
	a. Sensory: hyperalgesia (to pinprick) and/or allodynia (to light touch and/or deep somatic pressure and/or joint movement)	
	b. Vasomotor: temperature asymmetry and/or skin color changes and/or asymmetry	
	c. Sudomotor/edema: edema and/or sweating changes and/or sweating asymmetry	
	d. Motor/trophic: decreased range of motion and/or motor dysfunction (weakness, tremor, dystonia) and/or trophic changes (hair, nail, skin)	
	4. There is no other diagnosis that better explains the symptoms	

(continued on next page)

Table 2
(continued)

	Criteria or Distinguishing Features	Mechanism of Skin Findings
Small fiber neuropathy (SFN) with vasomotor symptoms[22]	1. Graded diagnostic criteria include clinical symptoms and objective testing: • Possible SFN: presence of length dependent symptoms and/or signs of small fiber damage • Probable SFN: presence of length dependent symptoms, signs of small fiber damage, normal sural nerve conduction study • Definitive SFN: presence of length dependent symptoms, signs of small fiber damage, normal sural nerve conduction study, low intraepidermal nerve fiber density at the ankle, and/or abnormal quantitative sensory testing (QSART) thermal thresholds in the foot. 2. Must exclude large fiber polyneuropathy with nerve conduction study or electromyography (EMG) 3. Must undergo skin biopsy or QSART to confirm SFN	Dysfunction of autonomic C fibers and small somatic sensory fibers which control blood vessel constriction and dilation as well as perception of pinprick and thermal stimuli
Achenbach syndrome[20]	1. Sudden blue discoloration of a digit (typically upper extremity) that is constant 2. May be minimally painful 3. Not typically cold to touch 4. Can occur in unusual locations like the proximal-mid digit rather than distal digit	Spontaneous venous hemorrhage

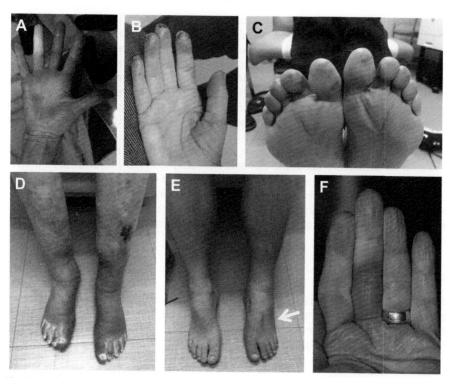

Fig. 2. Patients presenting with cold hands and feet: (*A*) patient with primary Raynaud's, experiencing all three phases of disease in the hands: pallor of the fourth digit, cyanosis of the fifth digit, and rubor of the third digit; (*B*) patient with SRP resulting in digital ulcerations in the setting of mixed connective tissue disease; (*C*) patient with bilateral reddish patches consistent with pernio of the feet; (*D*) elderly patient with acrocyanosis of the feet, using powder to counter hyperhidrosis; (*E*) young patient with Lisfranc injury of the left ankle resulting in vasomotor instability following surgery; and (*F*) patient with Achenbach syndrome or spontaneous venous hemorrhage of the third proximal digit. The *arrow* highlights skin discoloration and foot swelling in the affected limb. ([*A*] Image courtesy of Dr. Jeffrey Olin, Zena and Michael A. Wiener Cardiovascular Institute, Icahn School of Medicine at Mount Sinai.)

The distribution of symptoms and triggers is important to identify. RP typically affects the fingers and toes, although the nose, ears, or nipples can be affected. Thumb involvement is rare and is reported more frequently in patients with SRP.[23] Unilateral symptoms, or symptoms in a single affected limb, should raise suspicion for SRP. Secondary etiologies should be explored including occupational or hobby exposures (eg, vibratory injury, hypothenar hammer syndrome), medication or recreational exposures, associated signs and symptoms suggestive of underlying rheumatologic, infectious, or hematologic disease, family history of RP, and age at onset of symptoms (see **Table 1**).[24] Of note, although the mean age of onset for RP is in the mid-30s, SRP may present at any age.

The physical examination should be comprehensive with a focus on the vascular examination, including palpation of the radial, ulnar, brachial, dorsalis pedis, posterior tibial, popliteal, and femoral arteries bilaterally. The Allen test should be performed to detect any potential small vessel occlusion in the hand. Capillary refill should be assessed. The heart should be auscultated to detect any murmurs, arrhythmia, and the lungs for manifestations of interstitial pulmonary fibrosis associated with systemic sclerosis (SSc). The skin should be evaluated for any pitting, ulceration, sclerodactyly, skin thickening, calcinosis, or telangiectasias. If skin discoloration is present on examination, the affected area and distribution should be noted as well as any blanching or correction with raising the limb above the level of the heart (most suggestive of acrocyanosis). For patients without skin discoloration on examination, a request for photos of the discoloration events should be made so the patient can share their experience in full with the skilled provider.

tBeyond the history and examination, laboratory evaluation should be pursued to evaluate for secondary causes of patients with cold-induced vasospasm. At a minimum, basic testing is pursued as outlined in **Box 1**. If basic testing is positive, or if the patient presentation is suspicious for SRP, additional testing may be appropriate.[5] If the workup is negative, repeat testing should be considered with any worsening of symptoms or after 2 years of stable symptoms to determine if the patient has PRP.[6]

ADDITIONAL TESTING

Nailfold capillaroscopy is a useful tool for the identification of changes characteristic of patients with a scleroderma spectrum disorder in the setting of RP.[25] Nailfold videocapillaroscopy is the current gold standard and is increasingly used in everyday practice by clinical rheumatologists and research. A recent consensus statement was published to standardize the acquisition and analysis of data related to nailfold

---

Box 1
Laboratory testing for new or worsening symptoms of Raynaud phenomenon

Basic Evaluation
  Complete metabolic panel
  Complete blood count with differential
  Thyroid stimulating hormone
  Erythrocyte sedimentation rate
  C-reactive protein
  Urinalysis with urine sedimentation
  Antinuclear antibodies

Abnormal basic testing, or in patients with sclerodactyly, pitting, ulcerations
  Centromere antibodies
  Anti-topoisomerase I (SCL-70)
  Anti-ribonucleic acid (RNA) polymerase III
  Smith antibody
  Ribonucleioprotein (RNP)-antibody
  Phospholipid antibodies
  Lupus anticoagulant
  Beta-2 glycoprotein antibodies
  Cardiolipin antibodies
  Anti-Jo1
  Complement C3, C4
  Anti-double-stranded deoxyribonucleic acid (DNA) antibody
  Serum protein electrophoresis
  Cold agglutinins
  Cryoglobulins

capillaroscopy.[25] The premise of this technology is to detect early to late changes in the nailfold capillaries that indicate the presence of a scleroderma spectrum disorder (**Fig. 3**).[26]

Vascular testing may also be useful to distinguish reversible vasospasm from a fixed obstruction. Wrist brachial indices or ankle-brachial indices with digital pressures and digit photoplethysmography can provide useful information regarding digital perfusion.[27] These studies can be performed after warming to determine if an abnormality is reversible (**Fig. 4**). In some laboratories, cold immersion to bring out cold-induced vasospasm is performed, but we generally find this to be (1) painful for the patient and (2) unnecessary. The purpose of vascular testing is to identify fixed obstructions. Thus, if the physiologic study is normal at rest, it indicates that the patient does not have a fixed obstruction. Cold immersion testing is very sensitive for the presence of cold-induced vasospasm, but it is not specific and nearly half of the patients with a positive test do not have any symptoms of cold sensitivity.[28] The best correlate of symptoms with cold exposure remains a thorough history and physical examination as outlined above.

Rewarming in the presence of an abnormal physiologic test at rest, is useful to determine reversibility (and therefore may identify patients that will benefit from vasodilator medications as discussed in treatment options below). A normal digital systolic pressure is between 20 and 30 mm Hg of the brachial systolic pressure. Therefore, a normal digital brachial index (digital systolic blood pressure to brachial systolic blood pressure ratio) is considered greater than 0.8.[27] It is important to remember, however, that patients with distal ulceration may have normal digital-brachial indices because the digital cuff is placed around the proximal phalanx.

THERAPEUTIC OPTIONS

A detailed assessment and a log of RP triggers should be reviewed with the patient so that modifications may be made to avoid inciting factors. Conservative management, including maintenance of core body temperature with appropriate clothing is appropriate for all patients with RP.[3] All patients should be advised to avoid tobacco products and excess caffeine, as these agents enhance vasoconstriction.[29] Patients should also be counseled regarding safe rewarming procedures to avoid heat-induced injury in the setting of RP-induced anesthesia.[5] Local wound care instructions

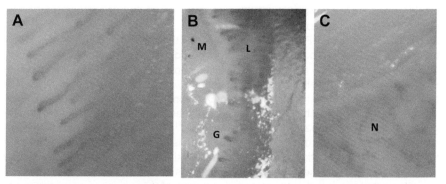

Fig. 3. Nailfold capillaroscopy demonstrating (*A*) normal capillaries, (*B*) active pattern with microhemorrhages (M), loss of capillaries (L), and giant capillaries (G), and (*C*) late pattern demonstrating neoangiogenesis (N). (Images courtesy of Dr. Lea Meir, Department of Rheumatology, Icahn School of Medicine at Mount Sinai.)

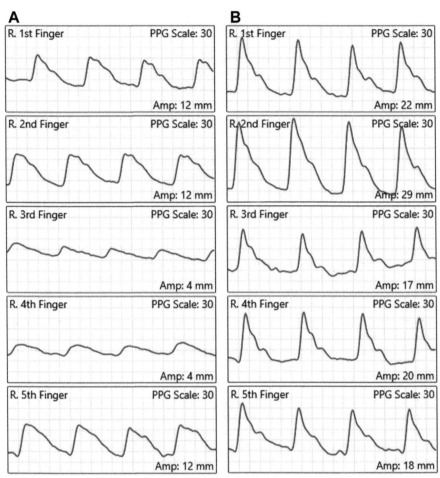

Fig. 4. Pulse volume recording (PVR) of the upper extremity digits demonstrating abnormal waveforms at rest (*A*), and normalization of all the PVR waveforms after rewarming (*B*).

should be reviewed with all patients with a wound. A general approach to the management of RP is summarized in **Fig. 5**.

Pharmacotherapy for RP targets the reduction of the number and frequency of Raynaud attacks. There is a paucity of high-quality randomized data. However, the available evidence supports non-cardioselective, long-acting dihydropyridine calcium channel blockers as first-line agents to reduce vasospasm.[30] It is important to note that RP is an off-label use for this class of medications. Alternatively, inhibitors of sympathetic tone with alpha-1 blockers have been studied in small randomized, cross-over studies and are a reasonable first choice as well.[31,32] It is recommended that treatment is initiated at a low dose of these medications and up-titrated to the treatment effect. Extended preparations should be used, starting with nifedipine ER 30 mg daily if a calcium channel blocker is used.[30,33] Prazosin is associated with dose-dependent side effects that are and should be started at a dose of 0.5 mg daily and up-titrated to treatment effect, over several days, to a maximum dose of 1 mg three times a day.[34]

Vasodilators are better studied in the management of SRP. A recent Cochrane review of patients with PRP determined that there was insufficient evidence to support

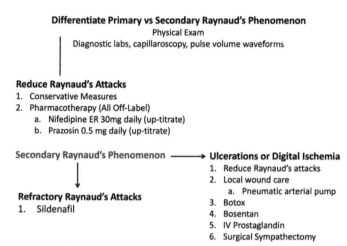

Differentiate Primary vs Secondary Raynaud's Phenomenon
Physical Exam
Diagnostic labs, capillaroscopy, pulse volume waveforms

Reduce Raynaud's Attacks
1. Conservative Measures
2. Pharmacotherapy (All Off-Label)
   a. Nifedipine ER 30mg daily (up-titrate)
   b. Prazosin 0.5 mg daily (up-titrate)

Secondary Raynaud's Phenomenon ⟶ **Ulcerations or Digital Ischemia**
1. Reduce Raynaud's attacks
2. Local wound care
   a. Pneumatic arterial pump
Refractory Raynaud's Attacks
1. Sildenafil
3. Botox
4. Bosentan
5. IV Prostaglandin
6. Surgical Sympathectomy

Fig. 5. Treatment algorithm for patients with RP.

the use of vasodilators, and the investigators concluded that vasodilators might even worsen disease.[35] In SRP related to SSc, however, phosphodiesterase-5 inhibitors (PDE5i) are considered first line in guideline-directed treatment of severe RP refractory to calcium channel blockers, or in patients with digital ulcerations.[36,37] One small randomized trial of 31 patients with SSc demonstrated a significant increase in digital ulcer healing with tadalafil 20 mg daily use on top of baseline vasodilator therapy. It also reported a reduced rate of new digital ulcer formation. A meta-analysis of three randomized trials including sildenafil 50 mg daily, sildenafil 100 mg increased to 200 mg daily, and tadalafil 20 mg daily reported increased rates of ulcer healing (relative risk [RR] 3.28, 95%confidence interval [CI] .32–8.13, $P < .01$) and improvement in ulcers when pooled data are compared with placebo (RR 4.29, 95%CI 1.73–10.66, $P < .002$).[38] The individual trials were not powered to detect a difference in ulcer healing. A second meta-analysis and systematic review of randomized data also determined an overall benefit in the frequency and severity of Raynaud's attacks with PDE-5 inhibition.[39] The Sildenafil Effect on Digital Ulcer healing in sClerodErma trial randomized patients to sildenafil 20 mg three times a day versus placebo over 12 weeks; there was no significant benefit in ulcer healing in patients receiving sildenafil.[40] Of note, the ulcer healing rate in the placebo was very high and the dose of sildenafil was lower than in previous trials included in the meta-analyses discussed above.

Alternative therapies beyond PDE5i include prostanoids (eg, intravenous iloprost) and endothelin-1 receptor agonists (eg, bosentan). Intravenous iloprost (0.5–2 ng/kg/min for 3–5 consecutive days) demonstrated a modest effect in the reduction of RP severity and attacks with benefit in ulcer healing for patients with SSc.[36–38] The oral prostanoids did not demonstrate a significant benefit, and intravenous iloprost remains unavailable in the United States.[38] One study of continuous intravenous epoprostenol (mean dose 2.2 ng/kg/min titrated up to mean dose 11.2 ng/kg/min over 12 weeks) for SSc patients with pulmonary arterial hypertension also demonstrated improvement in the severity of RP and reduced number of digital ulcers.[41] Adverse effects of prostanoids include headache, flushing, myalgias, nausea, and jaw pain.

The endothelin-1 receptor agonist, bosentan, has confirmed efficacy in high-quality randomized control trials to reduce the number of digital ulcers in patients with SSc.

The RAPIDS-2 trial compared bosentan (62.5 mg twice a day for 4 weeks, followed by 125 mg twice a day for 20 weeks) to placebo in 188 patients across 40 European centers.[42] Bosentan therapy resulted in a reduced number of new ulcerations at 6 months follow-up (mean 1.9 vs 2.7, $P = .04$). However, no difference in cardinal ulcer healing was observed between the two groups.[42] Guidelines recommend the addition of bosentan in patients with multiple digital ulcers despite the use of calcium channel blockers, intravenous prostanoids, or PDE5i.[36,37]

Less-supported therapies include serotonin reuptake inhibitors and angiotensin converting enzyme inhibitors, which demonstrated mild improvement in RP attack severity and frequency in patients with PRP.[43,44] Alternatively, topical agents to treat the localized vasospasm of Raynaud's attacks are attractive in patients that may not otherwise tolerate systemic vasodilators due to hypotension. Systematic reviews of topical nitrates suggest a moderate treatment effect in patients with SRP and a mild treatment effect for PRP.[45,46] Topical calcium channel blockers may not be as effective as topical nitrates, although further studies are needed.[47] A recent preclinical trial investigated a novel formulation of topical nifedipine that may be stable to UV-light, which has been a limitation of the utility for this drug in the past.[48] Topical PDE5i have also been investigated for the treatment of digital ulcerations in patients with SSc refractory to other therapies.[49] Future studies may identify a suitable topical therapy. However, the current data are overwhelmingly in favor of systemic therapies.

Pneumatic arterial pumps should be considered to assist with ulcer healing in patients with SRP. These devices cause intermittent venous occlusion, resulting in improved distal arterial perfusion and have demonstrated efficacy for wound healing and improved digital transcutaneous oxygen tension in patients with severe peripheral artery disease.[50] One study of 26 patients with upper extremity wounds secondary to SSc and thromboangiitis obliterans demonstrated complete healing of the ulceration in 96% with the use of a pneumatic arterial pump for 5 hours a day.[51] The mean time to wound healing was 22 weeks, and the mean duration of ulceration before treatment was 31 weeks. Most of the patients (25/26) noted improvement in pain with pump use.[51] Cost can be prohibitive for some patients, but the pneumatic arterial pump is an underused resource for patients with digital ulcers related to RP.

For patients who have failed all noninvasive therapies of RP, botulinum toxin A (10–100 units per hand) administered in the neurovascular bundle at the bifurcation of the common digital vessels is a promising therapy for refractory RP.[52–54] Botox preferentially inhibits cholinergic transmission. At low doses, it may inhibit acetylcholinergic vasodilation and sweating of the skin. At high doses, it inhibits sympathetic adrenergic vasoconstriction.[3] It also inhibits exocytosis of von Willebrand factor and endothelin-1, which play key roles in vasoconstriction and microthrombosis.[3] Historically, surgical sympathectomy was used for severe digital ulceration related to refractory RP with wide variability in reported techniques and results.[55]

SUMMARY

RP is an exaggerated response to cold stimuli that may be primary or secondary in etiology. The diagnosis is clinical and relies on thorough patient history and physical examination to distinguish RP from other small vessel vasomotor dysfunction such as acrocyanosis, pernio, SFN with vasomotor symptoms, and CRPS. Achenbach syndrome, which results from spontaneous venous hemorrhage in a digit, may also be mistaken due to the isolated discoloration but is a self-limiting phenomenon. Further evaluation with laboratory or vascular diagnostic laboratory testing may identify and clarify potential causes of SRP. The treatment of cold-induced vasospasm, regardless of etiology, is rooted in conservative warming techniques with avoidance of RP triggers and consideration of vasodilators, including calcium channel or alpha-1 blockers. More advanced SRP with digital ulceration may require PDE5i, endothelin-1 receptor blockers, and prostanoids. Refractory patients at risk for tissue loss with nonhealing wounds should consider pneumatic arterial pumps, botulinum toxin administration, or even surgical sympathectomy. More data are needed on the role of topical agents, including nitrates, calcium channel blockers, and PDE5i.

CLINICS CARE POINTS

- Raynaud's phenomenon (RP) refers to cold-induced vasospasm resulting in at least two phases of color change: pallor and cyanosis/rubor.
- Primary RP (Raynaud disease) is defined by (1) intermittent attacks with complete resolution, (2) bilateral findings, (3) absence of organic occlusion, (4) changes limited to the superficial skin, and (5) symptoms for at least 2 years with no other explanation.
- Laboratory testing may reveal secondary causes of RP and should be considered in patients with (see **Box 1**) abnormal basic testing and/or clinical clues on history of physical examination that point to a secondary cause (see **Table 1**).
- Nailfold capillaroscopy is increasingly used in rheumatology clinics and there is recent guidance on the appropriate use of this technology to evaluate patients with RP.
- Vascular testing with wrist-brachial indices and finger pressures with digit photoplethysmography may be performed at rest and with rewarming to determine if there is fixed obstruction present—this may allow for section of appropriate medical therapy and the identification of secondary disease.
- A reasonable approach to treatment includes avoidance of triggers with total body warming and initiation of calcium channel or alpha-1 blocker therapy in all patients with RP. Patients with SRP may additionally benefit from vasodilators (PDE5i, endothelin-1 receptor blockers, prostanoids), and pneumatic arterial pumps, botulinum-toxin therapy in the setting of nonhealing wounds and refractory RP.

DISCLOSURE

Speaker and teaching honorarium (Abbott Laboratories, Boston Scientific, Medscape, McGraw Hill), research funding (Philips Healthcare, NIH, United States RO1 HL148167 – The Define FMD Trial).

REFERENCES

1. Raynaud M. De l'asphyxie locale et de la gangrène symétrique des extrémités. 1862.
2. Herrick AL. The pathogenesis, diagnosis and treatment of Raynaud phenomenon. Nat Rev Rheumatol 2012;8(8):469–79.
3. Flavahan NA. A vascular mechanistic approach to understanding Raynaud phenomenon. Nat Rev Rheumatol 2015;11(3):146–58.
4. Cooke JP, Marshall JM. Mechanisms of Raynaud's disease. Vasc Med 2005; 10(4):293–307.
5. Choi E, Henkin S. Raynaud's phenomenon and related vasospastic disorders. Vasc Med 2021;26(1):56–70.
6. Allen EV, Brown JE. RAYNAUD'S DISEASE: A CLINICAL STUDY OF ONE HUNDRED AND FORTY-SEVEN CASES. JAMA 1932;99(18):1472–8.

7. Maverakis E, Patel F, Kronenberg DG, et al. International consensus criteria for the diagnosis of Raynaud's phenomenon. J Autoimmun 2014;48-49:60–5.

8. Stjernbrandt A, Pettersson H, Lundstrom R, et al. Incidence, remission, and persistence of Raynaud's phenomenon in the general population of northern Sweden: a prospective study. BMC Rheumatol 2022;6(1):41.

9. Rytkonen M, Raatikka VP, Nayha S, et al. [Exposure to cold and the symptoms thereof]. Duodecim 2005;121(4):419–23.

10. Silman A, Holligan S, Brennan P, et al. Prevalence of symptoms of Raynaud's phenomenon in general practice. BMJ 1990;301(6752):590–2.

11. Suter LG, Murabito JM, Felson DT, et al. The incidence and natural history of Raynaud's phenomenon in the community. Arthritis Rheum 2005;52(4):1259–63.

12. Spencer-Green G. Outcomes in primary Raynaud phenomenon: a meta-analysis of the frequency, rates, and predictors of transition to secondary diseases. Arch Intern Med 1998;158(6):595–600.

13. Creager MA, Perlstein TS, Halperin JL. Raynaud's Phenomenon. In: Creager MA, Beckman JA, Loscalzo J, editors. Vascular medicine: a Companion to Braunwald's heart disease. 2nd edition. Philadelphia: Elsevier Saunders; 2013. p. 587–99.

14. Garner R, Kumari R, Lanyon P, et al. Prevalence, risk factors and associations of primary Raynaud's phenomenon: systematic review and meta-analysis of observational studies. BMJ Open 2015;5(3):e006389.

15. Zahavi I, Chagnac A, Hering R, et al. Prevalence of Raynaud's phenomenon in patients with migraine. Arch Intern Med 1984;144(4):742–4.

16. Kurklinsky AK, Miller VM, Rooke TW. Acrocyanosis: the Flying Dutchman. Vasc Med 2011;16(4):288–301.

17. Olin JW. Vascular Diseases Related to Extremes in Environmental Temperature. In: Young JR, Olin JW, Bartholomew JR, editors. Peripheral vascular diseases. 2nd edition. St Louis (MO): Mosby-Year Book; 1996. p. 607–20.

18. Herman EW, Kezis JS, Silvers DN. A distinctive variant of pernio. Clinical and histopathologic study of nine cases. Arch Dermatol 1981;117(1):26–8.

19. Freeman EE, McMahon DE, Lipoff JB, et al. Pernio-like skin lesions associated with COVID-19: A case series of 318 patients from 8 countries. J Am Acad Dermatol 2020;83(2):486–92.

20. Yamamoto Y, Yamamoto S. Achenbach's Syndrome. N Engl J Med 2017; 376(26):e53.

21. Harden RN, McCabe CS, Goebel A, et al. Complex Regional Pain Syndrome: Practical Diagnostic and Treatment Guidelines, 5th Edition. Pain Med 2022; 23(Suppl 1):S1–53.

22. Zhou L. Small Fiber Neuropathy. Semin Neurol 2019;39(5):570–7.

23. Chikura B, Moore T, Manning J, et al. Thumb involvement in Raynaud's phenomenon as an indicator of underlying connective tissue disease. J Rheumatol 2010; 37(4):783–6.

24. Khouri C, Blaise S, Carpentier P, et al. Drug-induced Raynaud's phenomenon: beyond beta-adrenoceptor blockers. Br J Clin Pharmacol 2016;82(1):6–16.

25. Smith V, Herrick AL, Ingegnoli F, et al. Standardisation of nailfold capillaroscopy for the assessment of patients with Raynaud's phenomenon and systemic sclerosis. Autoimmun Rev 2020;19(3):102458.

26. Herrick AL, Cutolo M. Clinical implications from capillaroscopic analysis in patients with Raynaud's phenomenon and systemic sclerosis. Arthritis Rheum 2010;62(9):2595–604.

27. Moneta GL, Zacardi M. Noninvasive Diagnosis of Upper Extremity Arterial Disease. In: Zierler RE, editor. Strandness's Duplex Scanning in vascular disorders.

5th edition. Philadelphia, PA: Lippincott Williams & Wilkins, a Wolter Kluwer business; 2015. p. 172–82.

28. Porter JM, Snider RL, Bardana EJ, et al. The diagnosis and treatment of Raynaud's phenomenon. Surgery 1975;77(1):11–23.

29. Cardelli MB, Kleinsmith DM. Raynaud's phenomenon and disease. Med Clin North Am 1989;73(5):1127–41.

30. Rirash F, Tingey PC, Harding SE, et al. Calcium channel blockers for primary and secondary Raynaud's phenomenon. Cochrane Database Syst Rev 2017;12(12): CD000467.

31. Nielsen SL, Vitting K, Rasmussen K. Prazosin treatment of primary Raynaud's phenomenon. Eur J Clin Pharmacol 1983;24(3):421–3.

32. Wollersheim H, Thien T, Fennis J, et al. Double-blind, placebo-controlled study of prazosin in Raynaud's phenomenon. Clin Pharmacol Ther 1986;40(2):219–25.

33. Thompson AE, Pope JE. Calcium channel blockers for primary Raynaud's phenomenon: a meta-analysis. Rheumatology 2005;44(2):145–50.

34. Wollersheim H, Thien T. Dose-response study of prazosin in Raynaud's phenomenon: clinical effectiveness versus side effects. J Clin Pharmacol 1988;28(12): 1089–93.

35. Su KY, Sharma M, Kim HJ, et al. Vasodilators for primary Raynaud's phenomenon. Cochrane Database Syst Rev 2021;5(5):CD006687.

36. Kowal-Bielecka O, Fransen J, Avouac J, et al. Update of EULAR recommendations for the treatment of systemic sclerosis. Ann Rheum Dis 2017;76(8):1327–39.

37. de Vries-Bouwstra JK, Allanore Y, Matucci-Cerinic M, et al. Worldwide Expert Agreement on Updated Recommendations for the Treatment of Systemic Sclerosis. J Rheumatol 2020;47(2):249–54.

38. Tingey T, Shu J, Smuczek J, et al. Meta-analysis of healing and prevention of digital ulcers in systemic sclerosis. Arthritis Care Res 2013;65(9):1460–71.

39. Roustit M, Blaise S, Allanore Y, et al. Phosphodiesterase-5 inhibitors for the treatment of secondary Raynaud's phenomenon: systematic review and meta-analysis of randomised trials. Ann Rheum Dis 2013;72(10):1696–9.

40. Hachulla E, Hatron PY, Carpentier P, et al. Efficacy of sildenafil on ischaemic digital ulcer healing in systemic sclerosis: the placebo-controlled SEDUCE study. Ann Rheum Dis 2016;75(6):1009–15.

41. Badesch DB, Tapson VF, McGoon MD, et al. Continuous intravenous epoprostenol for pulmonary hypertension due to the scleroderma spectrum of disease. A randomized, controlled trial. Ann Intern Med 2000;132(6):425–34.

42. Matucci-Cerinic M, Denton CP, Furst DE, et al. Bosentan treatment of digital ulcers related to systemic sclerosis: results from the RAPIDS-2 randomised, double-blind, placebo-controlled trial. Ann Rheum Dis 2011;70(1):32–8.

43. Coleiro B, Marshall SE, Denton CP, et al. Treatment of Raynaud's phenomenon with the selective serotonin reuptake inhibitor fluoxetine. Rheumatology 2001; 40(9):1038–43.

44. Dziadzio M, Denton CP, Smith R, et al. Losartan therapy for Raynaud's phenomenon and scleroderma: clinical and biochemical findings in a fifteen-week, randomized, parallel-group, controlled trial. Arthritis Rheum 1999;42(12):2646–55.

45. Curtiss P, Schwager Z, Cobos G, et al. A systematic review and meta-analysis of the effects of topical nitrates in the treatment of primary and secondary Raynaud's phenomenon. J Am Acad Dermatol 2018;78(6):1110–8.e3.

46. Qiu O, Chan T, Luen M, et al. Use of nitroglycerin ointment to treat primary and secondary Raynaud's phenomenon: a systematic literature review. Rheumatol Int 2018;38(12):2209–16.

47. Wortsman X, Del Barrio-Diaz P, Meza-Romero R, et al. Nifedipine cream versus sildenafil cream for patients with secondary Raynaud phenomenon: A randomized, double-blind, controlled pilot study. J Am Acad Dermatol 2018;78(1): 189–90.

48. Wasan EK, Zhao J, Poteet J, et al. Development of a UV-Stabilized Topical Formulation of Nifedipine for the Treatment of Raynaud Phenomenon and Chilblains. Pharmaceutics 2019;11(11).

49. Fernandez-Codina A, Kazem M, Pope JE. Possible benefit of tadalafil cream for the treatment of Raynaud's phenomenon and digital ulcers in systemic sclerosis. Clin Rheumatol 2020;39(3):963–5.

50. Rooke TW, Osmundson PJ. Effect of intermittent venous occlusion on transcutaneous oxygen tension in lower limbs with severe arterial occlusive disease. Int J Cardiol 1988;21(1):76–8.

51. Pfizenmaier DH 2nd, Kavros SJ, Liedl DA, et al. Use of intermittent pneumatic compression for treatment of upper extremity vascular ulcers. Angiology 2005; 56(4):417–22.

52. Ennis D, Ahmad Z, Anderson MA, et al. Botulinum toxin in the management of primary and secondary Raynaud's phenomenon. Best Pract Res Clin Rheumatol 2021;35(3):101684.

53. Neumeister MW, Webb KN, Romanelli M. Minimally invasive treatment of Raynaud phenomenon: the role of botulinum type A. Hand Clin 2014;30(1):17–24.

54. Neumeister MW. The role of botulinum toxin in vasospastic disorders of the hand. Hand Clin 2015;31(1):23–37.

55. Coveliers HM, Hoexum F, Nederhoed JH, et al. Thoracic sympathectomy for digital ischemia: a summary of evidence. J Vasc Surg 2011;54(1):273–7.

Vasculitis: When to Consider this Diagnosis?

Kunal Mishra, DO, Randy K. Ramcharitar, MD,
Aditya M. Sharma, MD*

KEYWORDS

- Vasculitis • Diagnosis • Approach • Granulomatosis • Polyangiitis
- Takayasu arteritis • Giant cell arteritis

KEY POINTS

- Vasculitis is a diverse group of disorders involving inflammation of the blood vessels.
- Incorporating laboratory testing and imaging into a thorough clinical assessment is vital in identifying and diagnosing vasculitis.
- Vasculitis is a heterogeneous group of diseases with often adverse outcomes, and it will frequently require a multidisciplinary approach involving vascular medicine specialists, rheumatologists, and other specialties to provide good care.

INTRODUCTION

Vasculitis is a heterogeneous and complex group of disorders with the cardinal feature of inflammation of the blood vessels.[1] Diagnosis can be challenging, given diverse clinical presentations and varied organ involvement. In addition, treatment options are often complicated. It can be fatal if left untreated and often associated with significant long-term consequences and morbidities. This article reviews the key components an internist should be aware of in the diagnosis and care of patients with vasculitis.

CLASSIFICATION OF VASCULITIS

Vasculitis is classified into a primary or a secondary disorder. Primary is idiopathic, whereas secondary is often associated with an etiology such as infection, malignancy, and medications, to name a few.[1–3] Knowing which conditions or medications induce vasculitis is vital for physicians treating these disorders. These are outlined in **Box 1**. In addition, the presentation of the different types of vasculitis often overlap; hence, the diagnosis should never be made off one finding alone, and instead should be made by

Division of Cardiovascular Medicine, University of Virginia, 1215 Lee Street, PO BOX- 100058, Charlottesville, VA 22902, USA
* Corresponding author.
E-mail address: as8ah@uvahealth.org

Med Clin N Am 107 (2023) 845–859
https://doi.org/10.1016/j.mcna.2023.05.005
0025-7125/23/© 2023 Elsevier Inc. All rights reserved.

Box 1
Etiologies for secondary vasculitis

Infections:
  Viral: Hepatitis B and C, human immunodeficiency virus, parvovirus B19, cytomegalovirus, SARS-CoV-2, and herpes simplex virus.
  Bacterial: *Neisseria, Mycobacteria, Streptococcus, Salmonella, Staphylococcus, Clostridium septicum, Chlamydia pneumonia, Mycobacterium tuberculosis, Treponema pallidum, Borrelia burgdorferi, Cryptococcus, Neisseria,* and *Coccidioides.*
  Fungal: *Candida, Aspergillus,* and mucormycosis

Malignancies: Lymphoma, lymphoproliferative syndrome, acute myeloid leukemia, hairy cell leukemia, and so forth and also, solid organ tumors including lung, colon, and gastrointestinal (GI) malignancies.

Autoimmune and connective tissue disease: Relapsing polychondritis, Cogan syndrome, rheumatoid arthritis, Sjögren syndrome, systemic lupus erythematosus, scleroderma, primary biliary cirrhosis, and inflammatory bowel disease.

Medications: Penicillin, sulfa-drugs, allopurinol, thiazides, phenytoin, non-steroidal anti-inflammatory drugs (NSAIDs), quinidine, cocaine, heroin, amphetamines, propylthiouracil, hydralazine, minocycline, ciprofloxacin, pantoprazole, sulfonamides, and thiazides

Abbreviation: SARS-CoV-2, severe acute respiratory syndrome coronavirus 2.

---

a thorough review of clinical history, physical examination, laboratory and imaging findings, and sometimes biopsy results together, only then can the proper diagnosis i obtained and treatment be initiated.[2–4]

Vasculitis is subdivided based on primary vessel involvement as large-, medium-, and small-vessel vasculitis (LVV, MVV, and SVV) (**Box 2**). Large-vessel involvement includes the aorta and its major branches; medium vessels include renal and visceral

---

Box 2
Classification of vasculitides based on vessels involved

Large-vessel vasculitis
  Giant cell arteritis
  Takayasu arteritis
  Aortitis associated with spondyloarthropathies
  Idiopathic isolated aortitis and chronic periaortitis

Medium-vessel vasculitis
  Polyarteritis nodosa
  Kawasaki disease

Small-vessel vasculitis
  Immune complex vasculitis
    Cryoglobulinemic vasculitis
    Henoch–Schönlein purpura or IgA vasculitis
    Anti-glomerular basement membrane disease
  ANCA-associated vasculitis
    Eosinophilic granulomatosis with polyangiitis (Churg–Strauss syndrome)
    Microscopic polyangiitis
    Granulomatosis with polyangiitis (Wegener's granulomatosis)

Vasculitis involving arteries and veins of various sizes
  Behcet's syndrome
  Cogan syndrome

Abbreviations: ANCA, antineutrophil cytoplasmic antibody; IgA: immunoglobulin A.

---

arteries and veins and their branches. Small vessels often relate to arterioles, capillaries, and venules.[2–4] There is often an overlap in vessel involvement. **Box 2** provides a breakdown of different forms of vasculitic conditions based on the primary vessel involvement.

Large-Vessel Vasculitis

Giant cell arteritis (GCA), Takayasu arteritis (TA), and chronic periaortitis are the common forms of LVV.[3] LVV can often be seen in the form of secondary vasculitis, such as with relapsing polychondritis.

Clinical evaluation is the key. All patients suspected of LVV should undergo bilateral upper extremity blood pressure checks, cardiac auscultation, and assessment for vascular bruits or pulse differences in the carotid, temporal, and limb arteries. Laboratory testing will typically show elevated acute phase reactants (APR), such as elevated C-reactive protein or erythrocyte sedimentation rate. However, TA may not be associated with elevated APR even in its active state. Working through the diagnostic tree of LVV can be challenging, so it is important for a clinician to correctly use and interpret the clinical criteria, imaging, and at times, biopsy. Common imaging findings noted on duplex ultrasound, MRI, and computed tomography (CT) are a homogeneous, concentric thickening of the arterial wall in the acute stage (**Figs. 1** and **2**); however, aneurysms and stenoses can be seen in both active and chronic inactive stages.

Giant cell arteritis

Also called temporal arteritis is typically seen in adults older than 50 years, particularly above 70 years. Aorta and its branches are involved in, particularly carotid, ophthalmic, and temporal arteries[1,3] but can be seen in coronaries, renal and visceral arteries. Symptoms typically include headaches, visual impairment, and jaw claudication. Other systemic presentations are proximal arthralgia, fever, anemia, and fatigue. Monocular vision loss is the most feared acute complication of GCA; however, other serious complications of GCA include stroke, aortopathies, and limb ischemia. In an acute phase, elevated APRs are noted in most patients. The American College of Rheumatology (ACR) and the European League Against Rheumatism (EULAR) have released updated guidelines in 2022 for the diagnosis of LVV.[5] They provided a scoring system using clinical, laboratory, imaging, and biopsy results to classify GCA in a patient with LVV. This is outlined in **Table 1**.

Temporal artery biopsy has been a gold standard in diagnosing GCA. However, with recent imaging advances, EULAR now strongly recommends early imaging to

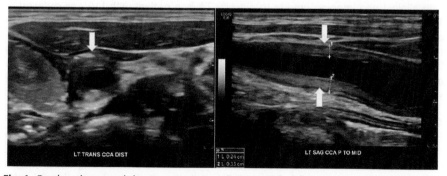

Fig. 1. Duplex ultrasound shows concentric wall thickening (*arrows*) along the left common carotid artery in a patient with active Takayasu arteritis.

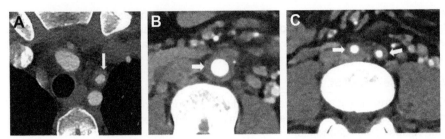

Fig. 2. Computed tomography angiogram shows concentric wall thickening (*arrows*) in the aorta (*B*) and its major branches [left common carotid; (*A*) and bilateral common iliac; *A* and C] arteries in patient with Takayasu arteritis.

complement the clinical diagnostic criteria for GCA. In patients with strong clinical suspicion for GCA with a positive imaging test, no additional test, such as a biopsy, is needed to diagnose GCA. Similarly, GCA diagnosis is unlikely in patients with low clinical probability and a negative imaging test. Temporal with axillary artery ultrasound is recommended as first-line imaging.[6] Additional tests such as MRI, CT, or PET may be used to detect wall inflammation or lumen changes in the arteries; however, this can be deferred to a specialist. Imaging is also instrumental when the recurrence of active disease is suspected in patients with a known history of LVV. Initial treatment is usually high-dose glucocorticoids with urgent referral to a vascular medicine specialist and or rheumatologist to assess for additional long-term steroid sparing therapies and long-term monitoring.[3]

Takayasu arteritis
A rare condition more reported in Asians; however, it has been found in other ethnicities and seen more frequently in women at the ages of 40 years or less.[1,7] It has similar vessels involved to GCA. The diagnosis of TA can be challenging due to nonspecific symptomatology such as arthralgias, intermittent fevers, and fatigue in the early stages. In addition, the insidious waxing and waning clinical course makes the diagnosis and management challenging. Brachial pulse deficits, blood pressure discrepancy, and limb claudication are critical characteristics but are not always specific to TA.[8] TA often leads to occlusions, stenoses, and ischemic damage to end organs, often leading to stroke, myocardial infarction, or renovascular hypertension.[9] The diagnosis of TA is often based on the summation of clinical characteristics, laboratory results, histopathology, and imaging. The 2022 guidelines provide a scoring system with clinical and imaging criteria to classify TA in a patient with LVV, as outlined in **Table 1**.[10] EULAR recommends MRI as first-line imaging to detect wall inflammation and or lumen changes in suspected TA.[6] A similar approach is recommended for long-term monitoring and assessment of recurrence of active disease, because APRs have limited use as they may be within the normal range even in the active phase of TA.[6] The initial treatment often involves glucocorticoids with referral to a specialist for long-term steroid sparing therapies and long-term monitoring.

Clinically isolated aortitis
Per the revised Chapel Hill vasculitis nomenclature, clinically isolated aortitis (CIA) is considered a single-organ vasculitis, given that it only impacts the aorta.[11] Initially, CIA can present with features consistent with infectious aortitis, granulomatosis with polyangiitis, or even GCA. CIA and GCA are histopathologically indistinguishable, but unlike GCA, CIA patients will typically not have cranial or inflammatory symptoms

Table 1
2022 updated American College of Rheumatology/European League against Rheumatism guidelines on classification of giant cell arteritis and Takayasu arteritis

ACR/EULAR Criteria for GCA Diagnosis		ACR/EULAR Criteria for Takayasu Arteritis	
Only Patients >50 can be Considered *Alternate Diagnoses Mimicking Vasculitis Should be Excluded First* *Only Apply this Criteria once Diagnosis of Large or Medium VESSEL Vasculitis has been made*		*Only Patients <60 can be Considered* *Patients MUST have Evidence of Vasculitis on Imaging*	
Clinical Criteria		*Clinical Criteria*	
Morning stiffness in shoulders/neck	+2	Female sex	+1
Sudden visual loss	+3	Angina/ischemic cardiac pain	+2
Jaw/tongue claudication	+2	Arm/leg claudication	+2
New temporal headache	+2	Vascular bruit (any large artery)	+2
Scalp tenderness	+2	Reduced pulse in upper extremity	+2
Abnormal examination of temporal artery (diminished pulse, tenderness, hard-cord-like appearance)	+2	Carotid artery abnormality (reduction/absence of pulse or tenderness)	+2
Laboratory/Imaging/Biopsy criteria		Systolic blood pressure difference in arms > 20 mmg	+1
Erythrocyte sedimentation rate >50 mm/h or C-reactive protein >10 mg/L	+3	*Imaging Criteria*	
Positive temporal artery biopsy or halo sign on temporal artery ultrasound	+5	Number of affected arterial territories (select one) One arterial territory Two arterial territories Three of more	+1 +2 +3
Bilateral axillary involvement	+2	Symmetric involvement of paired arteries	+1
FDG-PET activity throughout aorta	+2	Abdominal aorta involvement with renal or mesenteric involvement	+3
Add all the scores of the above 10 items if present. *A score of >6 points = Giant Cell Arteritis*		*Add all scores of above 10 items.* *A score >5 points = Takayasu Arteritis*	

Abbreviation: FDG-PET, fluorodeoxyglucose-PET.

with most patients presenting with cardiovascular symptoms such as dyspnea or chest pain. Most CIA patients tend to have aneurysmal dilation confined to the aorta with no evidence of wall thickening throughout the thoracoabdominal aortic wall. Treatment of most CIA patients of often surgical repair and given the lack of systemic inflammation, the use of corticosteroid treatment remains controversial.[11] Of note some studies show that even after surgical repair, CIA patients can continue to have aorta dilation, thus continued follow-up with either CTA or MRA is warranted.

Chronic idiopathic periaortitis
This is another LVV comprising inflammatory abdominal aortic aneurysm, retroperitoneal fibrosis, and perianeurysmal retroperitoneal fibrosis. Often seen in smokers and may present with chest, back, or abdominal pain. In cases of retroperitoneal fibrosis, it can also present with renal failure from ureteral obstruction.[12,13] However, patients can also be asymptomatic, with aortitis noted incidentally on imaging or

histopathology specimens after open aortic surgery. Treatment often includes immunosuppressive therapy.[12,13]

IgG4-related disease

This disease is characterized by findings or aortitis or periaortitis with elevated serum levels of IgG4.[3] Because biopsy is not always possible for these patients, imaging plays a significant role in diagnosing these patients. Most frequently the abdominal aorta is affected. The differential beyond other LVV when approaching IgG4-related disease (IgG4-RD) involving the aorta and retroperitoneum should be infectious etiologies such as syphilis. Steroids represent first-line therapy for these patients.[3]

Medium-Vessel Vasculitis

They have a broad range of clinical manifestations due to varied vascular and organ involvement. Polyarteritis nodosa (PAN) and Kawasaki disease (KD) are well-known MVV.

Polyarteritis nodosa

PAN is a necrotizing vasculitis associated with the characteristic appearance of microaneurysms in the renal (branch and intraparenchymal) and visceral arteries. Depending on vessel and organ involvement, the clinical presentation can be varied ranging from severe hypertension and renal insufficiency (kidneys), palpable purpura (**Fig. 3**), nodules, gangrene, pyoderma gangrenosum and livedo reticularis (see **Fig. 3**) (skin), arthralgias (musculoskeletal), abdominal discomfort, intestinal infarction and angina and gastrointestinal bleeding (gastrointestinal tract), sensory or motor neuropathies and mononeuritis multiplex (nervous system), and angina (cardiac).[14] APRs are elevated. PAN can be associated with hepatitis.[14] The initial treatment may involve glucocorticoids and cyclophosphamide; however, treatment is variable based on the disease type. PAN associated with hepatitis is treated with antiviral therapies, and hence, referral to a specialist is recommended for management.[14]

Kawasaki disease

It is primarily seen in young children presenting with myocarditis or endocarditis and is often associated with coronary aneurysms later in age.[15] Patients typically present with a fever for at least 5 days. American Heart Association guidelines on KD have noted the following as principal clinical features of KD: erythema and cracking of lips, strawberry tongue appearance and/or erythema of the oral and pharyngeal mucosa, bilateral conjunctival injection, skin rash, redness, and edema of the hand and

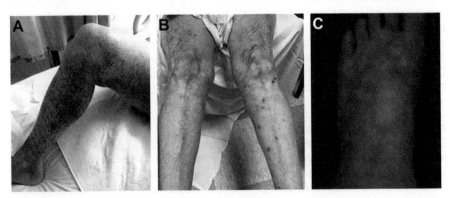

Fig. 3. (A) Palpable purpura and (B, C) livedo reticularis.

feet, and cervical lymphadenopathy.[15] The presence of prolonged fever and most of these features yields a substantial likelihood of KD. Initial tests include APR tests and echocardiogram. Treatment often includes aspirin and intravenous immunoglobulin. They may need treatment for coronary aneurysms later in age.

Small-Vessel Vasculitis

SVVs are further distinguished as antineutrophil cytoplasmic antibody (ANCA)-associated vasculitis (AAV) and immune complex SVV.

Antineutrophil cytoplasmic antibody-associated vasculitides

A necrotizing form of SVV with three major clinicopathologic types: granulomatosis with polyangiitis (GPA), microscopic polyangiitis (MPA), and eosinophilic GPA (EGPA).[1] Each of these is associated with circulating ANCA, the main target antigens being proteinase 3 (PR3) and myeloperoxidase (MPO). Also, there are patients with renal-limited AAV and ANCA-associated drug-induced vasculitis. There is controversy in differentiating MPA versus GPA as they share similar features with suggestions to classify based on antigen type rather than the traditional way. Clinical trials and research groups now classify AAV as MPO-ANCA versus PR3-ANCA. Mortality is higher in MPO-ANCA, and relapse rates are higher in PR3-ANCA. In 2022, the ACR and EULAR system developed a scoring system using clinical, laboratory, imaging, and biopsy criteria to classify AAV, which is noted in **Table 2**.[16–18]

AAV presents with a long insidious history of constitutional symptoms such as fever, myalgia, and fatigue with the exception of drug-induced. Cutaneous manifestations include nodules, palpable purpura, and ulcers (**Fig. 4**). GPA often demonstrates a triad of granulomatous inflammation and tissue destruction in the upper and lower airway and kidneys. Presentations include sinusitis, destructive rhinitis with the collapse of the nasal bridge and "saddle nose" deformity, and subglottic inflammation that may lead to tracheal stenosis.[19] Alveolar hemorrhage, venous thromboembolism, and inflammatory cardiac diseases are dangerous sequelae. Upper airway involvement is less common in MPA, which presents more with alveolar hemorrhage, scleritis, uveitis, skin lesions such as leukocytoclastic vasculitis (see **Fig. 4**), mononeuritis multiplex, and rapidly progressive glomerulonephritis.[19] Of note, glomerulonephritis is identical in both MPA and GPA. Mesenteric involvement may lead to abdominal pain and gastrointestinal bleeding. EGPA has the hallmark of asthma, significant peripheral eosinophilia, and systemic vasculitis manifestations in two or more extrapulmonary organs. EGPA has three phases: prodromal, eosinophilic, and vasculitic. The prodromal phase presents with asthma-associated diseases such as allergic rhinitis with or without polyposis. The eosinophilic phase, noted with eosinophilia, may be masked if steroids are used for asthma exacerbations. Pulmonary infiltrates, myocarditis, pericarditis, endocarditis, valvulitis, and coronary vasculitis have been reported in EGPA.[19] Renal manifestations are not as common as GPA or MPA.

Although most of these are serologically ANCA-positive, some of the patients are serologically ANCA-negative. Among GPA, 75% are PR3-ANCA, 20% are MPO-ANCA, and 5% are ANCA negative. Among MPA, 60% are MPO-ANCA, 30% are PR3-ANCA, and 10% are ANCA negative. Among EGPA, up to half are ANCA negative, and 45% are MPO-ANCA. Among renal-limited vasculitis and drug-induced vasculitis, up to 90% are MPO-ANCA, with less than 10% either PR3-ANCA or ANCA negative.[20] Glucocorticoids are the initial treatment of choice and may require additional advanced therapies.

Table 2
2022 updated American College of Rheumatology/European League against Rheumatism guidelines on classification of granulomatosis with polyangiitis, microscopic polyangiitis, and eosinophilic granulomatosis with polyangiitis

	Granulomatosis with Polyangiitis		Microscopic Polyangiitis		Eosinophilic Granulomatosis with Polyangiitis	
	Classification criteria should be applied to classify a patient as having GPA only when diagnosis of small- or medium-vessel vasculitis has been made		Classification criteria should be applied to classify a patient as having MPA only when diagnosis of small- or medium-vessel vasculitis has been made		Classification criteria should be applied to classify a patient as having EGPA only when diagnosis of small- or medium-vessel vasculitis has been made	
	Rule out mimics first		Rule out mimics first		Rule out mimics first	
Clinical Criteria						
Nasal involvement: ulcers, crusting, bloody discharge, congestion, blockage, or septal defect/perforation		+3	Nasal involvement: ulcers, crusting, bloody discharge, congestion, blockage, or septal defect/perforation	−3	Obstructive airway disease	+3
Cartilaginous involvement (inflammation of ear/nose cartilage, hoarse voice or stridor, endobronchial involvement or saddle nose deformity)		+2			Nasal polyps	+3
Conductive or sensorineural hearing loss		+1			Mononeuritis multiplex	+1
Laboratory/Imaging/Biopsy Criteria						
Pulmonary nodules, mass, or cavitation on chest imaging		+2	Positive test for pANCA or anti-MPO antibodies ANCA positive	+6	Blood eosinophil count $\geq 1 \times 10^9/L$	+5
Positive test for cytoplasmic antineutrophil cytoplasmic antibodies (cANCA) or antiproteinase 3 (anti-PR3) antibodies		+5	Fibrosis or interstitial lung disease on chest imaging	+3	Extravascular eosinophilic-predominant inflammation on biopsy	+2
Granuloma, extravascular granulomatous inflammation, or giant cells on biopsy		+2	Pauci-immune glomerulonephritis on biopsy	+2	Positive test for cANCA or anti-PR3 antibodies	−3
Inflammation, consolidation, or effusion of the nasal/paranasal sinuses or mastoiditis on imaging		+1	Positive test for cANCA or anti-PR3 antibodies	−1		
Pauci-immune glomerulonephritis on biopsy		+1			Hematuria	−1
Positive test for perinuclear antineutrophil-cytoplasmic antibodies (pANCA) or antimyeloperoxidase (anti-MPO) antibodies		−1	Blood eosinophil $\geq 1 \times 10^9/L$	−4		
Blood eosinophil count $\geq 1 \times 10^9/L$		−4				
	Sum the scores for 10 items, if present. A score of ≥ 5 is needed for classification of GPA		Sum the scores for 6 items if present. A score of ≥ 5 is needed for classification of MPA		Sum the scores for 7 items, if present. A score of ≥ 6 is needed for classification of EGPA	

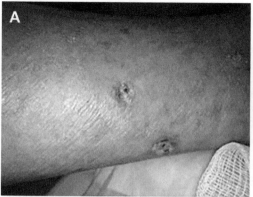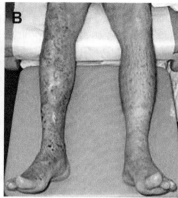

Fig. 4. (A) Ulcer in a patient with ANCA-associated vasculitis. (B) Leukocytoclastic vasculitis.

Immune complex small-vessel vasculitis

This includes cryoglobulinemic vasculitis, Henoch–Schönlein purpura (HSP), and anti-glomerular basement membrane (GBM) disease. HSP, called immunoglobulin A (IgA) vasculitis, presents with a triad of abdominal angina, inflammatory arthritis, and purpura.[21] Primarily seen in children and is characterized by IgA deposits in blood vessels. Renovascular hypertension caused by IgA glomerulonephritis is also seen, especially in children. Treatment is usually immunosuppressive therapy, depending on disease severity. Cryoglobulinemic vasculitis is often associated with hepatitis C but can occur with other chronic inflammatory diseases such as rheumatoid arthritis or lupus. Here, cryoglobulins induce immune-complex-mediated vasculitis presenting as arthralgias, myalgias, skin ulcerations, palpable purpura, glomerulonephritis, peripheral neuropathy, and renovascular hypertension, and Raynaud's phenomenon.[22] Laboratory tests show low complement levels and the presence of cryoglobulins. Skin biopsy reveals leukocytoclastic vasculitis for both HSP and cryoglobulinemic vasculitis.[21]

Last, anti-GBM disease, also called Goodpasture disease is caused by anti-basement membrane autoantibody deposition in the basement membrane of the pulmonary and glomerular capillaries. Manifestations are symptoms of alveolar hemorrhage and/or glomerulonephritis, along with the constitutional symptoms of SVV.[23] Often a renal biopsy is needed to clench the diagnosis.

Other Vasculitic Disorders and Presentations

Behcet disease

A chronic inflammatory disease involving both arteries and veins is seen more frequently in young people of Mediterranean, East Asian, and Middle Eastern descent. Manifestations include recurrent oral and/or genital aphthous ulcers and any of the following: skin lesions (erythema nodosum, pseudofolliculitis, and acneiform lesions), eye (uveitis and retinal vasculitis), neurologic (meningitis, stroke and cerebral venous thrombosis), musculoskeletal (intermittent symmetric oligoarticular arthritis), or gastrointestinal (melena, abdominal pain, and ulcerations) involvement.[24] Arterial complications include aneurysm, or rupture and venous complications are thrombosis. Immunosuppressive therapies are often the first line.

Single-organ vasculitis

Single-organ vasculitis is noted with vessels affected are limited to a single organ and has been discussed earlier for AAV-limited renal disease. However, it can involve other organs, including primary central nervous system vasculitis (CNSV), cutaneous SVV, isolated mesenteric vasculitis, and isolated aortitis. CNSV is seen in young-to-middle-aged adults affecting medium and small blood vessels of the brain, spinal cord, and the meninges. Manifestations are headache, stroke, seizures, aseptic meningitis, lethargy, and confusion.[25] Angiography will often show intracranial aneurysms and stenosis, which are hard to differentiate between other vascular disorders, and a multidisciplinary approach involving vascular specialists is helping in diagnosing CNSV.

Although cutaneous small vessel involvement is common in many forms of systemic vasculitis, isolated cutaneous SVV can occur and only present as palpable purpura, livedo reticularis or racemose, deep ulcers, or digital gangrene.[26] These are frequently drug or infection induced.

Mesenteric vasculitis usually occurs in conjunction with vasculitis of other organ systems, such as in PAN, TA, and Behcet disease; however, it can occur isolated in the form of single-organ vasculitis. Presentation is similar to ischemic colitis. Cross-sectional imaging can often help differentiate vasculitis from other forms of mesenteric vasculopathies, such as segmental arterial mediolysis, median arcuate ligament syndrome, and so forth. Emergent diagnosis is often necessary to avoid bowel ischemia and its complications.

Approach to Vasculitis

Stepwise approach to vasculitis

There are several vital steps in diagnosing and managing a patient with vasculitis. We recommend a stepwise approach.

Step 1: Think about vasculitis! Does the patient have signs and symptoms (including systemic and local) concerning vasculitis?

Step 2: Could this be a condition that mimics vasculitis?

Step 3: Secondary causes of vasculitis. Once mimics are ruled out, and there is a strong suspicion of vasculitis, could this be drug, infection or other condition inducing vasculitis?

Step 4: Identifying the type and extent of vasculitis: Do I need to do additional testing (laboratory, imaging, or histopathology)?

Step 5: Reduce or eliminate short-term complications. Do I need to treat with immunosuppressive therapy immediately before the specialist sees the patient?

Step 1: The first step for every clinician is to consider if the patient's presentation relates to vasculitis. In most cases of primary vasculitis, there is a prodromal phase of primarily constitutional symptoms lasting for weeks to months. Constitutional symptoms may include generalized fatigue, fever, malaise, weight loss, arthralgias, headaches, and myalgias. These may be associated with localized symptoms that could narrow down the specific vasculitic condition. Hence, a comprehensive history and physical examination are very vital. A complete vascular examination should take place to check for any pulse deficits and the presence of bruits. Pulmonary and cardiovascular examinations can also show the evidence of vasculitides, such as bruits noted in aortitis or pericardial rubs. A thorough skin examination to assess for findings of palpable purpura, macular lesions, livedo reticularis, oral, extremity, or genital aphthous ulcers, and peripheral cyanosis is essential (see **Figs. 3** and **4**). Although seeking to find the "worst" or most "well-known" manifestation of certain vasculitides may be necessary, having a broad view in a clinician's search is imperative not to have tunnel vision and ensure all clinical findings are noted.

Step 2: Several conditions can mimic vasculitis in their clinical presentation or imaging findings. Infection is a great masquerader of vasculitis. Vasculitis can lead to aneurysms, dissections, stenosis, occlusion, and rupture of the vessels; however, other vascular disorders such as fibromuscular dysplasia (FMD), atherosclerosis, and Ehlers–Danlos syndrome can lead to such findings. For example, PAN can be mistaken for FMD, a noninflammatory arteriopathy with microaneurysms presents more in the mid-distal sections of the main renal arteries.[27] However, unlike FMD, microaneurysms seem in the branch and intraparenchymal renal vessels in PAN. In addition, patients with PAN present with constitutional symptoms such as fever or arthralgias and high APRs, which are not seen in FMD.

Similarly, Ehlers–Danlos syndrome may have similar imaging findings of dissections, aneurysms, and stenosis such as vasculitis; however, these patients do not have inflammatory symptoms or elevated APR as seen in vasculitis, and they present with unique physical findings of hyperflexibility, delayed wound healing, and characteristic facial features. A multidisciplinary approach involving vascular medicine physicians and radiologists could be constructive in situations where the diagnosis is not precise. **Box 3** outlines common mimics of vasculitis.

Step 3: Once a strong clinical suspicion of vasculitis is established, mimics are ruled out. The patient should be evaluated for secondary causes of vasculitis. This can be achieved by assessing patients' medication history in addition to thorough history taking and physical examination, that is, could this be a drug-induced, recent infection-induced, or exposure-induced phenomenon? Drug history should include a history of prescription and over-the-counter drugs and illegal and herbal/alternative medicine products taken within the last year. Infection can be a mimic; however, can coexist

---

Box 3
Disorders mimicking vasculitis

Large-vessel vasculitis mimics
    Aortic aneurysms, including mycotic types
    Radiation-induced arteritis
    Atherosclerotic disease
    Inherited genetic connective tissue disorders: Marfan syndrome, Loeys–Dietz syndrome, and so forth
    Pseudoxantoma elasticum
    Coarctation of aorta and midaortic syndrome

Small- and medium-vessel vasculitis mimics
    Inherited genetic disorders noted in large-vessel vasculitis mimics
    Fibromuscular dysplasia
    Segmental arterial mediolysis
    Atherosclerotic disease noted in large-vessel vasculitis mimics
    Pseudoxanthoma elasticum noted in large-vessel vasculitic mimics
    Hypersensitivity reactions
    Infective endocarditis
    Disseminated intravascular coagulation
    Thrombotic thrombocytopenic purpura
    Antiphospholipid antibody syndrome
    Cholesterol embolization syndrome
    Vasospastic disease
    Atrial myxoma
    Vasoconstrictive drugs such as ergot and methysergide
    Reversible vasoconstriction syndrome
    Calciphylaxis
    Sickle cell disease
    Amyloidosis
    Moyamoya
    Radiation arteritis
    Systemic inflammatory conditions such as sarcoidosis or Susac syndrome

---

Box 4
Baseline laboratory investigations obtained when vasculitis is suspected

Complete blood count with differential

Acute phase reactants: Erythrocyte sedimentation rate and C-reactive protein

Renal and liver function test

Urinalysis

Pregnancy test is mandatory in female patients of child-bearing age

---

with vasculitis too, such as hepatitis B and C, and endocarditis and tuberculosis are some common ones. More recently, COVID-19 vasculitis has been noted frequently, which presents as cutaneous SVV and arterial and venous thrombosis.[28] Identification of secondary causes, as outlined in **Box 2**, is vital as treatment of vasculitis may significantly change in their presence. For instance, PAN associated with hepatitis B is treated initially with antiviral drugs rather than immunosuppressive therapy.[29] Drug-induced vasculitis may be treated only with discontinuation of the drug.[30]

Step 4: Identifying the extent of vasculitis is extremely important as it may change treatment. Evaluation for internal organ involvement in SVV to MVV and detailed vascular assessment in LVV to MVV should be strongly considered, especially in patients with evidence of ischemia, angiographic imaging studies such as computed tomography angiography (CTA) or MRA, or conventional angiograms should be considered to evaluate the extent of vascular involvement and potential consequences. Imaging can often help identify the extent of inflammation, particularly in LVV, as we note vessel wall thickening and edema on them (see **Figs. 1** and **2**). A PET scan is also helpful in identifying active inflammation.

Identifying the specific type of vasculitis often requires a combination of thorough clinical assessment, appropriate laboratory testing, and imaging. Imaging is beneficial in LVV and some MVV. For instance, a biopsy is not required to diagnose GCA in scenarios with strong clinical suspicion and positive imaging findings. However, inconclusive imaging findings may require a biopsy to prove the diagnosis. In addition, even when a biopsy is needed to confirm the diagnosis, imaging helps identify symptomatic organs, identifying the appropriate site for biopsy to improve the yield of results.

Box 4 notes blood tests often obtained when evaluating a patient for vasculitis. Checking renal function is essential as glomerulonephritis is a significant feature of many small–medium vessel vasculitides, with proteinuria or hematuria noted on the urinalysis.[5] In addition, eosinophilia is present in EGPA, GPA, or drug-induced vasculitis. Specific ANCA testing may help in the diagnosis of certain AAV. Similarly, testing for cryoglobulin or complement levels may be helpful when considering specific vasculitides.

Step 5: Certain vasculitides, if left untreated for some time, lead to severe complications. GCA, if untreated, can cause blindness or stroke. Identifying such scenarios and treating them with high-dose immunosuppressive therapies is vital even before the patient sees the specialist.

SUMMARY

Eyes do not see what the mind does not know—having a keen sense to consider the diagnosis of vasculitis when there are suspicious symptoms, even when nonspecific, is the first critical step. Incorporating laboratory testing and imaging into a thorough clinical assessment is vital in identifying and diagnosing vasculitis. Vasculitis is a heterogeneous group of diseases with often adverse outcomes, and it will frequently require a multidisciplinary approach involving vascular medicine specialists, rheumatologists, and other specialties to provide good care.

CLINICS CARE POINTS

- Vasculitis is a heterogeneous and complex group of disorders involving inflammation of blood vessels.

- The first step in diagnosing vasculitis will always be first to consider it does the patient have systemic and or local signs that may relate to a vasculitic process.

- Once vasculitis has been considered, it is essential to evaluate for mimics and secondary causes of vasculitis.

- Identify the type and extent of vasculitis; you can apply the 2022 American College of Rheumatology criteria to classify the type of vasculitis better.

- Once a diagnosis is made, try to limit any short-term complications; consider if the patient needs to be treated urgently with glucocorticoids before a specialist sees them.

DISCLOSURES

K. Mishra and R.K. Ramcharitar do not have any commercial or financial conflicts of interest and any funding sources to disclose. A.M. Sharma has institutional research grants from Vascular Medcure and Boston Scientific Corporation and received honorarium from Boston Scientific Corporation, United States.

ACKNOWLEDGMENTS

The authors would like to thank Drs Raghu Kolluri, Steven Dean, and Daniella Kadian-Dodov for providing **Fig. 4** (image A), **Fig. 4** (image B) and **Fig. 3** (image A), and **Fig. 1**, respectively.

REFERENCES

1. Jennette JC, Falk RJ, Bacon PA, et al. 2012 revised International chapel hill consensus conference nomenclature of vasculitides. Arthritis Rheum 2013; 65(1):1–11.
2. Sharma AM, Singh S, Lewis JE. Diagnostic approach in patients with suspected vasculitis. Tech Vasc Interv Radiol 2014;17(4):226–33.
3. Saadoun D, Vautier M, Cacoub P. Medium- and large-vessel vasculitis. Circulation 2021;143(3):267–82.
4. Suresh E. Diagnostic approach to patients with suspected vasculitis. Postgrad Med J 2006;82(970):483–8.
5. Ponte C, Grayson PC, Robson JC, et al. 2022 American college of rheumatology/EULAR classification criteria for giant cell arteritis. Arthritis Rheum 2022;74(12):1881–9.
6. Dejaco C, Ramiro S, Duftner C, et al. EULAR recommendations for the use of imaging in large vessel vasculitis in clinical practice. Ann Rheum Dis 2018;77(5):636–43.
7. Betrains A, Blockmans D. Diagnostic approaches for large vessel vasculitides. Open Access Rheumatol 2021;13:153–65.
8. Hellmich B, Agueda A, Monti S, et al. 2018 Update of the EULAR recommendations for the management of large vessel vasculitis. Ann Rheum Dis 2020;79(1): 19–30.

9. Tarkin JM, Gopalan D. Multimodality imaging of large-vessel vasculitis. Heart 2023;109(3):232–40.

10. Grayson PC, Ponte C, Suppiah R, et al. 2022 American college of rheumatology/ EULAR classification criteria for takayasu arteritis. Arthritis Rheum 2022;74(12): 1872–80.

11. Aghayev A, Bay CP, Tedeschi S, et al. clinically isolated aortitis: imaging features and clinical outcomes: comparison with giant cell arteritis and giant cell aortitis. Int J Cardiovasc Imaging 2021;37:1433–43.

12. Vaglio A, Buzio C. Chronic periaortitis: a spectrum of diseases. Curr Opin Rheumatol 2005;17(1):34–40.

13. Kuwana M, Wakino S, Yoshida T, et al. Retroperitoneal fibrosis associated with aortitis. Arthritis Rheum 1992;35(10):1245–7.

14. De Virgilio A, Greco A, Magliulo G, et al. Polyarteritis nodosa: a contemporary overview. Autoimmun Rev 2016;15(6):564–70.

15. McCrindle BW, Rowley AH, Newburger JW, et al. Diagnosis, treatment, and long-term management of Kawasaki disease: a scientific statement for health professionals from the American heart association. Circulation 2017;135(17): e927–99, published correction appears in Circulation. 2019 Jul 30;140(5): e181-e184.

16. Grayson PC, Ponte C, Suppiah R, et al. 2022 American College of Rheumatology/ European alliance of associations for rheumatology classification criteria for eosinophilic granulomatosis with polyangiitis. Ann Rheum Dis 2022;81(3):309–14.

17. Suppiah R, Robson JC, Grayson PC, et al. 2022 American College of Rheumatology/European alliance of associations for rheumatology classification criteria for microscopic polyangiitis. Arthritis Rheum 2022;74(3):400–6.

18. Robson JC, Grayson PC, Ponte C, et al. 2022 American College of Rheumatology/European Alliance of associations for rheumatology classification criteria for granulomatosis with polyangiitis. Ann Rheum Dis 2022;81(3):315–20.

19. Langford C. Clinical features and diagnosis of small-vessel vasculitis. Cleve Clin J Med 2012;79(Suppl 3):S3–7.

20. Geetha D, Jefferson JA. ANCA-associated vasculitis: core curriculum 2020. Am J Kidney Dis 2020;75(1):124–37.

21. McCarthy HJ, Tizard EJ. Clinical practice: diagnosis and management of Henoch-Schönlein purpura. Eur J Pediatr 2010;169(6):643–50.

22. Lamprecht P, Gause A, Gross WL. Cryoglobulinemic vasculitis. Arthritis Rheum 1999;42(12):2507–16.

23. Kluth DC, Rees AJ. Anti-glomerular basement membrane disease. J Am Soc Nephrol 1999;10(11):2446–53.

24. Yurdakul S, Hamuryudan V, Yazici H. Behçet syndrome. Curr Opin Rheumatol 2004;16(1):38–42.

25. Byram K, Hajj-Ali RA, Calabrese L. CNS vasculitis: an approach to differential diagnosis and management. Curr Rheumatol Rep 2018;20(7):37.

26. Loricera J, Blanco R, Ortiz-Sanjuán F, et al. Single-organ cutaneous small-vessel vasculitis according to the 2012 revised International Chapel Hill Consensus Conference Nomenclature of Vasculitides: a study of 60 patients from a series of 766 cutaneous vasculitis cases. Rheumatology 2015;54(1):77–82.

27. Gornik HL, Persu A, Adlam D, et al. First International Consensus on the diagnosis and management of fibromuscular dysplasia. Vasc Med 2019;24(2): 164–89, published correction appears in Vasc Med. 2019 Oct;24(5):475] [published correction appears in Vasc Med. 2021 Aug;26(4):NP1.

28. McGonagle D, Bridgewood C, Ramanan AV, et al. COVID-19 vasculitis and novel vasculitis mimics. Lancet Rheumatol 2021;3(3):e224–33.
29. Guillevin L, Mahr A, Callard P, et al. Hepatitis B virus-associated polyarteritis nodosa: clinical characteristics, outcome, and impact of treatment in 115 patients. Medicine (Baltim) 2005;84(5):313–22.
30. Cuellar ML. Drug-induced vasculitis. Curr Rheumatol Rep 2002;4(1):55–9.

Unprovoked Venous Thromboembolism
The Search for the Cause

Hunter Mwansa, MBBS, Mohamed Zghouzi, MD,
Geoffrey D. Barnes, MD, MSc*

KEYWORDS

- Unprovoked venous thromboembolism • Evaluation • Recurrence risk assessment
- Thrombophilia • Anticoagulation

KEY POINTS

- An index VTE event without identifiable risk factors (unprovoked VTE) has a higher recurrence risk than VTE associated with major transient risk factors.
- Most patients with unprovoked VTE require secondary thromboprophylaxis upon the completion of the primary treatment phase if they have no high bleeding risk.
- Risk prediction models can help identify patients at low VTE recurrence risk who may discontinue anticoagulation upon the completion of the primary treatment phase.
- Avoid routine thrombophilia testing in patients with unprovoked VTE.

INTRODUCTION

Venous thromboembolism (VTE) is a common vascular disorder encompassing deep vein thrombosis (DVT) and pulmonary embolism (PE).

EPIDEMIOLOGY

There is no data on global estimates of VTE prevalence and incidence. In the US, approximately 1,015,000 people had VTE in 2018, with PE accounting for 38% of cases.[1] The annual incidence of VTE in six European countries (total population 310.4 million) was 762,000 in 2007, with PE accounting for 39% of cases.[2] The incidence of VTE is lower in Australia and South Korea compared to the US and Europe (0.8 vs 0.2 vs 1–2 per 100-person years, respectively).[3] There is limited data on VTE incidence in the developing world. In the US, the overall lifetime risk of VTE at 45 years is 8.1%, and this risk is higher among Black individuals (11.5%), particularly those of

Frankel Cardiovascular Center, University of Michigan, Ann Arbor, MI, USA
* Corresponding author. Frankel Cardiovascular Center, 1500 E. Medical Center Drive, Ann Arbor, MI 48109.
E-mail address: gbarnes@med.umich.edu

Med Clin N Am 107 (2023) 861–882
https://doi.org/10.1016/j.mcna.2023.05.006
medical.theclinics.com

low socioeconomic status.[4] Further, VTE incidence increases with age and is eight-fold higher in individuals $\geq$80 years compared to those aged 50 years.[5] The relationship between VTE incidence and biological sex varies with age, with premenopausal women having a higher age-adjusted incidence than men.[3] This likely reflects the higher VTE risk in reproductive-age women, which is likely multifactorial.[6]

VTE incidence has increased, with PE accounting for a greater proportion of VTE among the elderly.[1] VTE imposes substantial morbidity, mortality, and economic costs in healthcare and lost productivity years.[1] A multinational computerized registry found VTE-related mortality of 2.6% for lower extremity DVT, 3.31% for upper extremity DVT, and 5.13% for PE within 30 days of diagnosis.[7] In the US, the financial cost of VTE is over $1.5 billion per year.[1]

Venous thromboembolism risk factors

VTE involves the formation and propagation of blood clots within deep veins. It is due to the disruption of normal blood components and venous function due to a complex interplay of vascular injury, venous stasis, and hypercoagulability.[8] Intrinsic patient-specific VTE risk factors and/or acquired environmental or non-environmental provoking factors influence VTE risk.[3,8] About 20% of VTE events are cancer-associated, 20% to 30% have transient risk factors (**Table 1**), while 40% to 50% have no identifiable provoking factors.[9] Previously, VTE was categorized into "provoked" and "unprovoked" VTE based on the presence or absence of acquired VTE provoking factors. While important in guiding VTE recurrence risk assessment and duration of anticoagulant therapy, this dichotomization of VTE has significant limitations. First, there is inconsistency in the distinction between "provoked" and "unprovoked" VTE in clinical practice and research studies. Second, there can be overlapping and/or existence of multiple VTE risks within the same individual. Third, there is heterogeneity in VTE recurrence risk even among patients within the same VTE category.[10,11] As such, more recent VTE guidelines[12,13] emphasize individualized VTE risk assessment in lieu of dichotomized VTE categorization. However, "Unprovoked" VTE will be used given its widespread adoption and use to achieve this chapter's learning objectives.

Briefly, intrinsic/independent VTE risk factors are patient-specific factors including age greater than 50 years, male sex, tall stature, non-O ABO blood group, obesity, race/ethnicity, left iliac compression syndrome, family history, and hereditary thrombophilia. Setting-related or acquired VTE risks are factors associated with VTE if they are present within 2 to 3 months of the index VTE event.[14] These risks are either surgical or nonsurgical and can further be divided into minor transient, major transient, minor persistent, and major persistent risk factors based on their reversibility and strength of association with VTE incidence (see **Table 1**). This conceptual framework has major implications on VTE recurrence risk, prognosis, and anticoagulant therapy. Patients with surgical major transient/reversible risk factors at the time of the index VTE event have the lowest annualized VTE recurrence risk (1.0% per patient-year), while those with nonsurgical transient provoking factors have a higher annualized VTE recurrence risk (5.8% per patient-year) after the discontinuation of time-limited anticoagulation (see **Table 1**; **Table 2**).[15,16] The likelihood of recurrent VTE and death is higher in patients with VTE associated with weak transient-provoking factors than in patients with major transient-provoking factors.[10]

Persistent major VTE risk factors (active cancer and cancer therapy) are associated with the highest risk of VTE recurrence [20.7% versus 6.8% for cancer versus non-cancer associated VTE, respectively; hazards ratio 3.2].[13,17] Patients with VTE without identifiable provoking factors have an intermediate annualized recurrence risk 7.9% after the discontinuation of time-limited anticoagulation.[15]

Table 1
Venous thromboembolism (VTE) risk factor categorization

[a]Major Transient/Reversible Risks	[b] Minor Transient/Reversible Risks	Minor Persistent Risks	Major Persistent Risks
• [c]major surgery with anesthesia ≥30 min • Cesarean section • [d]major trauma • hospitalization for acute illness with attendant immobility for ≥3 d) • [e]COVID-19 infection	• hospitalization <3 d for acute illness and/or without immobility • laparoscopic surgery • minor leg trauma with transient immobility • flight >8 h • OCP/HRT/IVF • pregnancy and puerperium	• non-malignant persistent risks (eg, active IBD and autoimmune diseases, eg, Lupus, Rheumatoid arthritis) • history of VTE in first-degree relative or known minor thrombophilia • renal impairment (CrCl <50mL/min) • Heart failure • nephrotic syndrome • chronic indwelling venous catheters (eg, dialysis) and cardiac device lead wires • Lower extremity paralysis or paresis • age≥50 y • obesity (BMI≥30 Kg/m²) • chronic venous insufficiency, including varicose veins	• [f]active cancer and/or ongoing cancer therapy

Abbreviations: BMI, body mass index; HRT, hormone replacement therapy; IBD, inflammatory bowel disease; IVF, in-vitro fertilization; OCP, estrogen-containing contraceptive.

[a] Provoking factors present within 3 mo of index VTE.

[b] Provoking factors present within 2 mo of index VTE.

[c] Variable risk but generally higher for orthopedic surgery and neurological surgery.[86]

[d] Variable risk but higher in patients with spinal cord injury or spinal fractures with paralysis, head injury, pelvic fractures, lower extremity long-bone fractures, trauma-related bone fracture, operatively treated bone fractures, venous injury.[86]

[e] COVID-19, coronavirus-2019 requiring hospitalization (risk higher for critically ill patients)[87]

[f] Variable risk depending on cancer type, stage, patient race/ethnicity, and cancer therapy (higher VTE risk in pancreatic, brain, lung, ovarian, and metastatic cancer; highest risk in Black individuals; increased risk with myeloma therapy, antiangiogenic, and antiestrogen therapy)[88].

Table 2
Risk factors for recurrent VTE after stopping anticoagulants[92]

Risk Factors	Risk ratio[a]
Major transient risk factor vs unprovoked	0.2
Minor transient risk factor vs unprovoked	0.5
Cancer vs unprovoked	1.5–3
Noncancer persistent risk factor	1.5–2
Isolated distal DVT vs proximal DVT	0.2–0.5
Proximal DVT vs PE without proximal DVT	1.4
Previous VTE: yes vs no	1.5
Male vs female (after unprovoked VTE)	1.75
Elevated d-dimer (after unprovoked VTE): yes vs no	1.5–2.5
Antiphospholipid antibody: yes vs no	1.5–3
Hereditary thrombophilia: yes vs no	1.2–2.0
Asian vs white or black	0.8
Residual DVT on ultrasound	1.4

Abbreviations: DVT, deep vein thrombosis; PE, pulmonary embolism; VTE, venous thromboembolism.
[a] As the influence of risk factors on the risk for recurrence may not be independent, the overall risk ratio associated with a combination of factors may not be the product of the individual risk ratios.
Data from [Kearon C, Kahn SR. Long-term treatment of venous thromboembolism. *Blood.* Jan 30 2020;135(5):317-325. doi:10.1182/blood.2019002364] with permission.

"Unprovoked venous thromboembolism"

The occurrence of a VTE event in the absence of identifiable provoking factors has previously been termed "unprovoked" VTE. Therefore, the characterization of VTE as "unprovoked" requires the exclusion of acquired transient and persistent provoking factors. Despite variation in individual patient risk for recurrent VTE after a first episode of unprovoked VTE,[10] most patients have higher recurrence rates after stopping time-limited anticoagulants.[10] In patients with a first unprovoked VTE who completed at least 3 months of anticoagulation, cumulative recurrence rates after stopping antico-agulation were 10% at 1 year, 16% at 2 years, 25% at 5 years, and 36% at 10 years.[11]

Unprovoked venous thromboembolism recurrence risk assessment
Predictors of venous thromboembolism recurrence. VTE recurrence risk depends on the presence or absence of VTE-provoking factors and the nature of these provoking factors (see **Tables 1** and **2**) if present at the time of the index VTE event. Other factors known to influence VTE recurrence risk include elevated D-dimers, location of VTE (distal vs proximal DVT or PE), male sex, age less than 50 years at index VTE, and post-thrombotic syndrome (see **Tables 1** and **2**; **Table 3**). VTE recurrence risk assessment can be challenging because of risk variability among patients with unprovoked VTE.

Venous thromboembolism recurrence risk prediction tools. Several models to aid VTE recurrence risk quantification in patients with unprovoked VTE exist (see **Table 3**). However, it is essential to recognize that these recurrent risk prediction tools have methodological limitations and have modest predictive performance in external validation studies.[18] Thus, they may underestimate or overestimate VTE recurrence risk and must be applied with caution.[18] The HERDOO2 and Vienna scores have good

Table 3
Unprovoked VTE recurrence risk prediction models

Prediction Model	Risk Predictive Variables	Low-Recurrence Risk categories[a]	Population Studied	Study Type
DASH	• D-dimer$\geq$500 ng/mL after stopping anticoagulation • Age<50 y • Male Sex • Hormonal therapy	• Score $\leq$1	Unprovoked VTE or VTE with minor risk factors	Retrospective patient-level meta-analysis
DAMOVES	• Abnormal D-dimer during anticoagulation • Age per 10 y increase • Mutation (heterozygous FVL and/or prothrombin G20210A) • Obesity with BMI>30Kg/m^2 • Varicose veins • Factor Eight (VIII) activity • male Sex	Score <11.5 according to nomogram (0–30 points) [b]	Unprovoked VTE	Prospective cohort
[e]HERDOO2	• D-dimer$\geq$250 ng/mL before stopping AC • Age $\geq$65 y • BMI $\geq$30Kg/m^2 • Hyperpigmentation, edema, redness	Score = 0–1 point	Unprovoked VTE or VTE with minor risk factors	Prospective cohort
[d]L-TRRiP (model C)	• Male sex • Popliteal DVT • Proximal DVT • PE and DVT • Surgery prior to index DVT • DVT related to pregnancy/puerperium • Hormone use at VTE onset • Plaster cast prior to index VTE	2-y predicted VTE recurrence risk 0%–32%	Provoked and unprovoked VTE	Population-based case-control study

(continued on next page)

Table 3
(continued)

Prediction Model	Risk Predictive Variables	Low-Recurrence Risk categories[a]	Population Studied	Study Type
	• Immobilization in bed prior to VTE onset • History of CVD • Blood group O vs non-O • FVL			
Vienna	• D-dimer after stopping anticoagulation • Male sex • VTE location (distal DVT, proximal DVT, PE)	Low risk if score ≤180 according to nomogram[c]	Unprovoked VTE	Prospective cohort

Abbreviations: AC, anticoagulation; BMI, body mass index; CVD, cardiovascular disease; DVT, deep vein thrombosis; FVL, Factor V Leiden; PE, pulmonary embolism; VTE, venous thromboembolism.

DASH score ≤1 corresponds to annualized VTE risk of 3.1% (95% CI, 2.3%-3.9%).

[a] VTE recurrence risk considered low if ≤ 5% per International Society of Thrombosis and Hemostasis recommendation.[89]

[b] DAMOVES score less than 11.5 corresponds to annualized VTE recurrence less than 5%[90].

[c] Low risk corresponds to annualized VTE recurrence risk of 4.4% (95% CI, 2.7%-6.2%).

[d] L-TRRiP, Leiden Thrombosis Recurrence Risk Prediction.[91]

[e] Can reliably identify female patients with a low annualized risk of 3% (95% CI, 1.8%-4.8%) for VTE recurrence after a first episode of unprovoked VTE; among all men and high-risk women with HERDOO2 score≥2 those who discontinued anticoagulation, the annualized VTE recurrence risk was high 8.1% (95% CI, 5.2%-11.9%)[18].

to excellent predictive accuracy in identifying patients at low risk for recurrent VTE after a first unprovoked VTE (see **Table 3**). The HERDOO2[18] can identify female patients at low risk for recurrence after a first unprovoked VTE in whom anticoagulants can safely be discontinued after 3 months. While these risk prediction tools can also identify patients with high VTE recurrence risk, their utility in managing high-risk patients after a first unprovoked VTE is limited since such patients require extended anticoagulation if bleeding risk is not prohibitively high. Cancer-specific recurrent risk prediction models are beyond the scope of this article.[19,20]

Venous thromboembolism presentation, evaluation, and management

Clinical presentation
Patients with upper extremity or lower extremity DVT usually present acutely with non-specific asymmetric extremity swelling, warmth, redness, and pain. Patients with acute PE may present with non-specific symptoms, including acute onset dyspnea, cough, hemoptysis, pleuritic chest pain, palpitations, lightheadedness, near syncope, and syncope. At times, VTE is diagnosed incidentally on imaging done for other indications. History should therefore aim to elicit VTE symptoms, focusing on pertinent positives and negatives, as well as VTE risk factors (see **Table 1**). Inquiry on systemic manifestations, constitutional symptoms, rash, skin discoloration, arthralgias, chronic diarrhea, eye symptoms, ischemic events, spontaneous abortions, premature deliveries, pre-eclampsia, in-vitro-reproductive therapies, gender-affirming hormonal treatments, family history of VTE, gender- and age-specific cancer screens, autoimmune conditions, and malignancy may help uncover VTE predispositions in patients with what might initially appear unprovoked VTE.

Physical examination
A focused physical exam may reveal asymmetric limb edema with erythema and tenderness. Massive extremity edema, cyanosis, extremity coldness with diminished and/or absent pulses, and impaired motor/sensory function must alert the clinician of limb-threatening ischemia due to phlegmasia. Patients with PE may have respiratory distress, hypoxia, low-grade fever, tachycardia, hypotension, jugular venous pressure elevation, accentuated pulmonary component of P2, and cold extremities if in cardiogenic shock. The presence of symmetrical hand synovitis, lupus rash, livedo reticularis, livedo racemosa, lymphadenopathy, nodules, and masses may suggest potential underlying diseases.

Investigations
The initial evaluation of a patient depends on clinical presentation, VTE risk factors, and the pretest probability of VTE. Evaluation and management of patients with high-risk PE or high-likelihood PE presenting with hemodynamic instability are beyond the scope of this article. Multiple clinical prediction models exist to aid the determination of the pretest probability of VTE, but the most widely used are the Geneva and Wells score (**Table 4**). The Pulmonary Embolism Rule-out Criteria (PERC) developed to rule out PE in emergency department patients with low clinical probability for PE is also available. The PERC criteria comprise eight variables significantly associated with an absence of PE (age<50 years; heart rate <100 beats/min; oxygen saturation >95% on room air; no unilateral leg swelling; no hemoptysis; no recent trauma nor surgery requiring general anesthesia within 4 weeks; no prior VTE; no hormone use in both men and women). The use of the PERC rule in very low-risk emergency department patients can safely exclude PE and reduce health costs due to decreased computed tomography (CT) utilization and quicker discharges.[21] The PERC must be applied cautiously as it can miss PE in 8% of patients with low pretest probability.

Table 4
Clinical assessment of VTE pretest probability

Geneva score[92]		Wells Score for PE[93]		Wells Score for DVT[93]	
Variables	Points	Items	Points	Variables	Points
Previous DVT/PE	3	Previous objectively diagnosed DVT/PE	1.5	Paralysis, paresis, or recent plaster immobilization of leg	1
Heart rate 75–94 bpm	3			Bedridden recently for >3 d or surgery within the last 12 wk	1
Heart rate ≥95 bpm	5	Heart rate>100bpm	1.5	Localized tenderness along the deep venous system	1
Surgery or fracture within the past month	2	Immobilization≥3 d or surgery within the past 4 wk	1.5	Entire leg swollen	1
Hemoptysis	2	Hemoptysis	1	Non-varicose collateral superficial veins	1
Active cancer	2	Malignancy with treatment within 6 mo or palliative therapy	1	Calf>3cm compared to other leg	1
Unilateral lower limb pain	3	Clinical signs and symptoms of DVT	3	Pitting edema confined to symptomatic leg	1
Pain on lower-limb deep venous palpation and edema	4	PE is #1 diagnosis or just equally likely	3	Prior history of confirmed DVT	1
Age≥65 y	1			Active malignancy	
				Alternate diagnosis to DVT as likely or more likely	−2
Clinical probability					
3-level score					
Low	0–3		<2		<1
Intermediate	4–10		2–6		1–2
High	≥11		>6		>2

Fulfilling the PERC requires the absence of all PERC items in patients with a low pretest probability of PE.

The Geneva and Wells scores were derived and validated to assess the clinical pretest probability of VTE. Both tools have simplified versions that are validated and available online. Based on the clinical pretest score (see **Table 4**), the probability of DVT or PE is determined. Patients with a high pretest probability for DVT or PE require confirmatory imaging with compression ultrasonography or CT pulmonary angiography (CTPA) [lung perfusion scintigraphy if CTPA contraindicated], respectively. Patients with low and intermediate pretest probability for DVT/PE require additional testing with a moderate or high sensitivity D-dimer to improve the pretest probability of VTE. A negative moderate or high-sensitivity D-dimer is usually sufficient to exclude VTE in most patients with low to intermediate pretest probability because of its high negative predictive value.[22] However, D-dimer increases with advancing age[23] resulting in diminished negative predictive value in elderly patients. In the ADJUST-PE prospective validation study, the use of optimal age-adjusted D-dimer level (patient's age at 50 years or greater x 10) compared to a fixed D-dimer $\geq$500 ng/mL in patients with low and intermediate clinical pretest probability of PE resulted in a larger number of patients in whom PE could safely be excluded without additional false positives.[24] Patients with low to intermediate DVT/PE probability in whom a moderate to high-sensitivity D-dimer is elevated warrant further evaluation with imaging.

Evaluation of pulmonary embolism. CTPA is the diagnostic test of choice for confirmation of PE. If CTPA is contraindicated, lung perfusion (V/Q) scintigraphy has reasonable diagnostic accuracy, particularly in patients with normal chest radiographs. V/Q lung scans combine lung ventilation and perfusion assessments using radiotracers. Lung perfusion is abnormal, while ventilation is normal in patients with acute PE. V/Q lung scans pick perfusion defects in areas of normal lung ventilation (mismatch). Trinary V/Q lung reporting results include high probability (considered diagnostic in most patients), non-diagnostic, and normal scan (excludes PE). High clinical suspicion for PE and the presence of a proximal DVT on compression ultrasonography and/or a right heart thrombus is sufficient to diagnose PE if CTPA and lung scintigraphy are not feasible.[25] Chest x-rays are usually abnormal but non-specific for PE but can help exclude other differentials such as pneumonia and flash pulmonary edema. The most common ECG abnormality in PE is sinus tachycardia. Other ECG findings more specific for right ventricular strain in severe PE include the classic but rare S1Q3T3 pattern (S wave in lead I, Q wave in lead III, inverted T wave in lead III), T wave inversions in leads V1-V4, and a QR pattern in V1. ECG may also help exclude other differentials, such as ST-elevation myocardial infarction. Cardiac biomarkers (troponin I, BNP, and NT-proBNP) and transthoracic echocardiography help assess the presence of right ventricular strain and dysfunction as well as right heart thrombi which are essential in PE risk stratification. Integrating multiple clinical variables, including echocardiography, cardiac biomarkers, and multivariable PE risk stratification tools such as the pulmonary embolism severity index and Bova scores, can help predict 7-day and 30-day mortality in patients with acute PE.[26]

Evaluation of deep vein thrombosi. Compression ultrasonography helps confirm DVT in patients with high clinical pretest probability and patients with low to intermediate pretest probability who also have positive moderate to high-sensitivity D-dimers. If the clinical suspicion for DVT remains high despite a negative compression ultrasound result, repeating compression ultrasonography in 7 to 10 days is recommended to help confirm or exclude DVT.[16] CT venography or MR venography are reasonable considerations for DVT diagnosis when pelvic or ilio-caval thrombosis is suspected. These should be suspected in patients with severe bilateral lower extremity symptoms, non-compressive deep proximal veins with no identifiable thrombus, and loss of respiro-phasicity on spectral Doppler waveforms.

Evaluation for occult malignancy. VTE risk is higher in patients with cancer,[27] and there is an increased likelihood of cancer diagnosis in patients in whom VTE is unprovoked.[28] However, unselected extensive evaluation for occult malignancy in patients with unprovoked VTE without symptoms, signs, or laboratory abnormalities suggestive of cancer is not associated with improved survival.[28] This approach leads to increased healthcare costs and patient morbidity, including anxiety.[28,29] A strategy incorporating limited evaluation focused on a thorough review of the patient's history, physical exam, basic laboratory (complete blood count, calcium, hepatic function test, urinalysis), chest radiographs, gender- and age-appropriate cancer screens (breast, cervical, colorectal, prostate) is recommended when evaluating patients with unprovoked VTE for occult malignancy.[28,29] However, patients with unprovoked VTE who have concurrent clinical findings suspicious of malignancy warrant directed cancer evaluation based on their clinical presentation.[28,29]

Thrombophilia. Thrombophilia refers to hereditary and/or acquired conditions associated with increased predisposition to thrombosis. It may be challenging to distinguish between hereditary and acquired thrombophilia due to their complex interplay.[30] A perturbed homeostatic balance between procoagulant and anticoagulant proteins results in hypercoagulability. Therefore, thrombophilia may result from increased procoagulant activity or decreased anticoagulant activity. Examples of thrombophilia due to increased procoagulant activity include factor V Leiden and prothrombin gene mutation G20210A.[31,32] Thrombophilia resulting from a decreased anticoagulant activity is far less common and includes protein C, protein S, and antithrombin III deficiency.[33]

Inherited thrombophilia

Factor V Leiden mutation Accounts for the most common inherited thrombophilia leading to increased resistance of activated protein C (APC).[34] Mutation in the gene encoding for factor V (G1691A) results in the inability of APC to degrade factor V. This phenomenon in the setting of other VTE risk factors heightens VTE risk. Heterozygous FVL is present in about 3% to 10% of Caucasians, but less common in other races and ethnic groups.[35] It exhibits autosomal dominance inheritance.[36] Individuals with heterozygous FVL mutation can have a four-fold higher VTE risk compared to unaffected individuals.[37] The screening test is the activated protein C assay, which, if positive is confirmed by genetic testing.[38]

Prothrombin mutation G20210A A gene located on chromosome 11 encodes for prothrombin protein and substitution of G to A on nucleotide position 20,210 at 3' untranslated region of the gene. The mutation increases prothrombin levels in the blood and VTE risk.[39,40] The mutation prevalence in the general population is about 3%, mainly in Caucasians, and is associated with a three-fold increase in VTE risk.[37] It is transmitted in an autosomal dominant fashion and diagnosed by DNA testing.[41]

Protein C deficiency Protein C is a vitamin K-dependent anticoagulant protein. Vitamin K facilitates the gamma-carboxylation of N-glutamic acid residues in the liver.[42] Heterozygous Protein C deficiency has a prevalence of 1.5% in the general population.[43] It is associated with a 2 to 11-fold higher risk of VTE.[44] More than 270 different mutations have been linked to protein C deficiency.[45] These mutations can cause a decreased synthesis of the protein (Type I) or the synthesis of a malfunctioning molecule (Type II).[46] It exhibits autosomal dominance inheritance. Heterozygosity may result in mild protein C deficiency. Patients who are homozygous or compound heterozygous may exhibit more severe disease.[47] Protein C deficiency is diagnosed using protein C assays.[48] Testing should be avoided in conditions associated with acquired protein C deficiency (eg, acute thrombosis, using vitamin K antagonists, or liver disease) to avoid false test results.

Protein S deficiency Protein S is another vitamin K-dependent protein synthesized in the liver. Circulating protein S is either bound to complement protein (60%) or free (40%).[49] Protein S serves as a cofactor for APC, which facilitates the inactivation of factors Va and VIIIa. It also serves as a tissue factor pathway inhibitor leading to a decrease in thrombin formation.[50,51] Protein S deficiency exhibits autosomal dominance inheritance.[52] It is found in less than 0.1% of the general population. Patients with protein S deficiency have a 2.4 increased fold risk of VTE.[53] Quantitative defect (Type I and III) are more common, while qualitative defects (Type II) are rare.[54] Diagnosis of protein S deficiency can be difficult due to variability in testing assays. Assays available for evaluating protein S deficiency are the activity, free antigen, and total antigen assays. The recommended approach requires screening with the free antigen assay followed by the activity assay for the confirmation of the diagnosis in patients with an abnormal screen.[55]

Antithrombin deficiency Antithrombin (AT) exerts its anticoagulant effects by inhibiting activated thrombin, factor X, and IX. Heparin accelerates AT activity. It is a rare thrombophilia and is usually inherited as autosomal dominant.[56] Its prevalence in the general population is 0.02% to 0.17%, but has a prevalence of 0.5% to 4.9% in patients with VTE.[57] Mutation in the gene SERPIN1 causes antithrombin deficiency; more than 250 variations in the mutation have been described. AT deficiency can be quantitative (Type I) or qualitative (Type II). Further, three subtypes of type II have been recognized, with one due to a heparin-binding side defect, which is of clinical importance as heterozygous carriers of such mutations have lower risks of thromboembolic disease. There are two antithrombin assays, functional (activity) and immunoassay (antigen). Initial testing with the activity assay followed by the antigen assay to determine the type of deficiency is the recommended approach.[58]

Acquired thrombophilia
Antiphospholipid syndrome Circulating antiphospholipid antibodies [aPL (Lupus anticoagulant, immunoglobulin G or M anticardiolipin, and anti-Beta-2 glycoprotein I)] underpin the pathophysiologic process of APS. Recurrent thrombosis is most strongly associated with the Lupus anticoagulant (LA), but the presence of all three antibodies (triple positive) elevates recurrence risk. The estimated incidence and prevalence of APS in the general population is 5 and 50 per 100,000, respectively.[59] About 50% of patients with SLE have aPL.[60] Thrombotic APS is associated with recurrent thrombosis, neurological symptoms, and recurrent abortions in women.[61] Rarely, patients may present with life-threatening multiorgan failure due to extensive microvascular thrombosis when they have catastrophic APS. Other causes of elevated aPL include chronic diseases, inflammation, or acute infection. Vitamin K antagonists (VKAs) and direct-Xa inhibitors can also cause falsely positive LA. The revised Sapporo criteria can help ascertain the significance of positive aPL results and APS diagnosis (**Table 5**).[62] Patients diagnosed with APS usually require lifelong anticoagulation. VKAs are the recommended therapy for triple-positive APS. It is crucial to understand that PT is affected in patients with lupus inhibitors. Therefore, the use of chromogenic factor X therapeutic level is essential in ascertaining therapeutic INR in such patients.[63]

Table 5 summarizes APS diagnostic criteria	
Clinical criteria[a]	1. Vascular thrombosis (arterial/venous/microvascular).
	2. Pregnancy morbidity (unexplained fetal loss beyond 10th weeks of gestation / 3 or > spontaneous abortions before 10 weeks of gestation / premature birth before 34th weeks due to eclampsia or insufficiency of the placenta.
Laboratory criteria[b]	1. Lupus anticoagulant (LA) present in plasma.
	2. Anticardiolipin (aCL) antibody IgG and/or IgM (>40 GPL or MPL, or >the 99th percentile).
	3. Anti-β2 glycoprotein-I antibody IgG and/or IgM (in titer >the 99th percentile)

[a] One clinical and one laboratory criterion are needed to establish the diagnosis of APS.
[b] Laboratory criteria need to be present on two or more occasions more than 12 wk apart.

Testing for thrombophilia One or more thrombophilia can be identified in about 50% of all patients with unprovoked VTE. VTE at young age less than 50 with recurrence, strong family history of VTE at age less than 50, and thrombosis in unusual sites (cerebral veins and splanchnic) may help identify patients likely to have underlying thrombophilia.[64–67] Risk for a first VTE event is elevated in patients with thrombophilia, but data on whether thrombophilia elevates VTE recurrence risk is less clear.[68]

Testing for thrombophilia is performed routinely despite recommendations that testing be performed only in patients in whom results may have management implications. Thrombophilia testing can be offered in appropriately selected patients with unprovoked VTE if results will impact anticoagulant choices, as in patients with triple-positive APS, and if it can inform the primary prevention of VTE in asymptomatic family members of the patient. The use of DOACs in patients with triple-positive APS and APS associated with microvascular thrombosis is associated with an increased risk of arterial thrombosis (LMWH-bridged VKA recommended over DOACs).[69] Knowledge of underlying thrombophilia may influence decisions regarding hormonal therapy and oral contraception in female relatives of the affected patient. Unselected thrombophilia testing is associated with high healthcare costs and patient anxiety.[70] Appropriate patient selection is key in mitigating unintended consequences of routine testing.[71]

Thrombophilia testing does not usually affect the duration of anticoagulant therapy in patients with unprovoked VTE. Testing for FVL, G20210A mutation, AT deficiency, and aPL (except for LA) is feasible at the time of VTE diagnosis. Testing for other thrombophilia during the acute phase of VTE and while on anticoagulation may lead to false positives. Anticoagulants should be stopped for a minimum of 5 days in patients receiving VKAs or 2 to 3 days if receiving DOACs.

Methylenetetrahydrofolate reductase (MTHFR) gene variants are associated with elevated homocysteine levels but have no clear association with VTE risk.[72,73] Thus, testing for MTHFR deficiency in patients with VTE is unnecessary and costly.

Venous thromboembolism management
Acute management of PE in patients with hemodynamic instability or high-risk PE, intermediate-risk PE, and limb-threatening extremity DVT is beyond the scope of this article. Suffice to say that such emergencies require timely multidisciplinary care, including pulmonary embolism response teams (PERT)[12] to guide patient management.

For most patients with VTE, anticoagulation is the mainstay of therapy. Initiation of anticoagulation hinges on the balance of risks (bleeding complication) and benefits (decreased VTE recurrence), patient preferences, and costs of medications. Anticoagulant management can broadly be divided into 3 phases—initial treatment phase (7–21 days), during which time patients are rapidly initiated on intense anticoagulation with either parenteral or higher doses of oral anticoagulants to disrupt active thrombosis and prevent clot propagation, primary treatment phase (3–6 months after initial phase) which mitigates VTE recurrence given the high recurrence risk during 3 to 6 months, and extended phase for secondary VTE prevention beyond the primary phase with no defined timely.[8,74] VTE recurrence risk falls rapidly after the initiation of anticoagulation, then gradually falls before the attainment of a new baseline and relatively stable recurrence risk in 3 to 6 months while on anticoagulation.[74,75] Extended anticoagulation decreases recurrent VTE risk by 80% to 90% but is associated with increased bleeding complications (3%–4% annualized risk of major bleeds with VKAs).[12,13,76] Recurrent VTE has a cumulative incidence of 36% at 10 years after stopping anticoagulants compared to a 12% risk of major bleeding from extended therapy.[11] However, major bleeding is associated with a 2-3-fold higher risk of death than recurrent VTE (fatality of 4% and 11% from recurrent VTE and major bleeding, respectively).[12,13,77] Head-to-head comparative studies of VKAs and direct-acting oral anticoagulants (DOACs) showed that DOACs are non-inferior to VKAs and are associated with a 40% lower risk of major bleeding complications, including intracranial bleeds.[12,77–79] Higher bleeding complications reported from rivaroxaban and edoxaban use in cancer-associated VTE were primarily driven by gastrointestinal and urothelial malignancies.[80] Low-dose DOACs are effective in secondary VTE prevention and are associated with lower bleeding risk.[79] The efficacy of low-dose DOACs for secondary VTE prevention in high-recurrence risk patients (eg, recurrent unprovoked VTE, cancer-associated VTE) has not been investigated.[81] Earlier meta-analyses on DOACs must be interpreted cautiously as more contemporary meta-analyses suggest smaller differences in major bleeding complications between VKA and DOACs than previously reported.[79,82] AC-related bleeding events are highly variable and depend to a considerable extent on individual patient characteristics and clinical setting.[74,75] Further, there is currently no bleeding risk prediction tool with good predictive accuracy and validation to aid the quantification of bleeding risk.[18] As such, most guidelines recommend extended therapy in patients with high recurrent VTE risk after a first unprovoked VTE only if the patient's bleeding risk is low to moderate.[12,13,25] The use of clinical gestalt to assess individual patients' bleeding risk is recommended. The ACCP's proposed bleeding risk assessment is stratified into low risk (no risk factors; 0.8%/year risk of major bleeding), moderate risk (1 risk factor; 1.6%/year risk of major bleeding), and high risk (≥2 factors; 6.5%/year risk of major bleeding).[12] Factors to consider when using the ACCP's suggested bleeding risk assessment include advanced age (age>65; worse for age>75), prior bleeding, especially if uncorrected, thrombocytopenia, anemia, prior stroke, cancer (greater risk for highly vascular and metastatic cancers), alcohol abuse, liver failure, renal insufficiency, diabetes, hypertension, concomitant antiplatelet and NSAID use, reduced functional capacity, frequent falls, and poor control of vitamin K antagonist therapy.[12] **Table 6** gives a synopsis of guideline recommendations on managing patients with unprovoked VTE in specific clinical scenarios.

Anticoagulant therapy. During the initial treatment phase, patients eligible for anticoagulation can be treated with either parenteral or higher-dose oral anticoagulants. Multiple factors influence the choice of anticoagulant during the initial treatment phase including clinical setting (inpatient care with acute medical/surgical needs vs outpatient care), medical comorbidities (eg, renal and liver dysfunction), and patient preferences.

Table 6
Guideline recommendations on the management of specific unprovoked VTE clinical scenarios

Unprovoked VTE Clinical Scenario	Guideline Recommendations on the Management of Unprovoked VTE in Specific Clinical Scenarios				
	ACCP 2021 Guidelines[12]	ASH 2020 Guidelines[81]	2nd Consensus Document on Diagnosis and Management of DVT (ESC Working Groups) 2021[13]	ESC 2019 PE Guidelines[25]	NICE 2020 Guidelines[29]
First unprovoked VTE (proximal DVT and/or PE)	Extended therapy for most patients[c]	Extended therapy for most patients[c]	Extended therapy for most patients[c]	Extended therapy for most patients[c]	Extended therapy for most patients[c]
Recurrent VTE	Extended therapy[c]	Extended therapy[c]	Extended therapy[c]	Extended therapy[c]	Extended therapy[c]
[a]IDDVT in patients with risk factors for thrombi extension or higher recurrence risk[b]	Manage just like proximal DVT and/or PE (no specific guidance on extended therapy)	No specific guidance	Manage just like proximal DVT and/or PE (no specific guidance on extended therapy)	Not applicable	No specific guidance
ISSPE and no proximal DVT	Manage just like proximal DVT and/or PE in patients at elevated risk for recurrence if CTPA findings suggest a true-positive result[d]	No specific guidance	Not applicable	ESC guidelines emphasize the interpretation of CTPA findings in the context of clinical pretest probability for PE given a high PPV value of CTPA (92%–96%) and low PPV (58%) in patients with low to intermediate clinical pretest probability for PE, respectively[16]	No specific guidance

Unprovoked VTE with elevated risk for recurrence who refuse extended AC	Aspirin 100 mg daily if not contraindicated	Aspirin 100 mg daily if not contraindicated	No specific guidance	No specific guidance	Aspirin 100–150 mg daily if not contraindicated
Unprovoked proximal DVT and/or PE in patients with active bleeding and/or progressive or recurrent VTE while on AC[e]	IVC filter placement	IVC filter placement	IVC filter placement	IVC filter placement	IVC filter placement

Abbreviations: AC, anticoagulant/anticoagulation; ACCP, American College of Chest Physicians; ASH, American Society of Hematology; CTPA, computed tomography pulmonary angiography; ESC, European Society of Cardiology; IDDVT, isolated distal deep vein thrombosis; ISSPE, isolated subsegmental pulmonary embolism; IVC, inferior vena cava; NICE, National Institute for Health and Care Excellence; PPV, positive predictive value; VTE, venous thromboembolism.

[a] Deep lower extremity vein thrombosis with most proximal extent distal to the popliteal vein.

[b] Risks for extension and/or recurrence include "unprovoked DVT" or persistent VTE risks, elevated D-dimer, bilateral lower extremity thrombi, thrombi involving greater than 1 calf vein, thrombi greater than 5 cm in length and/or greater than 7 mm in diameter, highly symptomatic patient.[12]

[c] Refers to patients with low to moderate bleeding risk.

[d] CTPA findings suggestive of true positive PE: good opacification of distal pulmonary arteries; multiple intraluminal defects; defects involving more proximal subsegmental arteries; centrally located filling defects (surrounded by contrast rather than adherent to vessel wall); high clinical pretest probability for PE.[12]

[e] Consider IVC filter retrieval and anticoagulation if the patient no longer has a contraindication to anticoagulation—cause of bleeding addressed in patients with reversible causes of bleeding.

Commonly available anticoagulants for the initial treatment phase include unfractionated heparin (UFH), low-molecular-weight heparin (LMWH), heparin-bridged VKA, and factor-Xa-inhibitors.

UFH's rapid onset of action and quick systemic clearance make it a favorable anticoagulant in hospitalized patients requiring invasive procedures. Heparin-induced thrombocytopenia (HIT) can complicate UFH therapy. Weight-adjusted LMWH is another parenteral option with rapid onset of action, more predictable anticoagulant effects, lower risks for HIT, and longer duration of action than UFH. It can be administered once or twice daily depending on a patient's body mass and renal function. LMWH also requires less monitoring than UFH. However, patients with renal dysfunction and extremes of body weight may require anti-factor-Xa levels for efficacy and safety reasons. Direct thrombin inhibitors Argatroban and Bivalirudin are options in patients with a history of HIT and/or who develop HIT while on heparin.

Factor-Xa-inhibitors (apixaban and rivaroxaban) are also favorable options for initial VTE management at higher doses (apixaban 10 mg twice daily for 7 days; 5 mg twice daily thereafter; rivaroxaban 15 mg twice daily for 21 days; 20 mg daily). Other DOACs (dabigatran and edoxaban) require a parenteral lead-in with either UFH or LMWH for 5 to 10 days before the initiation of therapy. Unlike heparin-bridged VKA, which runs concurrently with parenteral therapy, dabigatran, and edoxaban are usually started after the completion of the parenteral lead-in. Apixaban and rivaroxaban appear more convenient because they do not require frequent laboratory monitoring in eligible patients who prefer the oral-only anticoagulant strategy, provided there are no contraindications and cost-prohibitive insurance co-pays. Heparin-bridged VKAs, including acenocoumarin, phenprocoumon, and warfarin are also an option for the initial treatment phase. Bridging VKA with heparins is essential to prevent prothrombotic VKA complications related to functional deficiencies of vitamin K-dependent clotting factors (II, VII, IX, Xa) and anticoagulant proteins C and S. The concurrent administration runs for at least 5 days and is usually maintained for 24 to 48 hours after the attainment of a therapeutic international normalized ratio (INR) of 2.0 to 3.0 (target 2.5). VKAs have a narrow therapeutic index and significant variability among patients warranting frequent monitoring for efficacy and safety reasons. They also have significant food- and drug-drug interactions. Therefore, most guidelines now recommend DOACs over VKAs for eligible patients as first-line VTE therapy.

Assess for potentially provoking risk factors Most patients in whom VTE occurs in the absence of transient/reversible VTE-provoking factors at the time of the index VTE have an elevated risk of recurrence and benefit from extended anticoagulation if their bleeding risk is not high.

Reassessment of the patient for reversible or persistent VTE risks is critical when deciding to stop or extend anticoagulation after the primary treatment phase is completed. The patient's VTE recurrence risk must outweigh their bleeding risk to achieve a favorable net clinical benefit from extended anticoagulation. It is essential to identify VTE complications, bleeding complications, and other new conditions (eg, renal dysfunction, hepatic dysfunction, significant changes in weight, dietary changes, medication changes with potential drug-drug interactions) which may influence decisions regarding extended anticoagulation, choice of anticoagulant as well as dosages. The 3-month mark is also an opportunity to repeat compression ultrasonography to establish a new baseline in patients with index proximal DVT with a high clot burden in whom this baseline comparison serves to identify recurrent DVT in the future if anticoagulation is discontinued.

Recommend extended treatment for most patients without a reversible risk factor if bleeding risk is not prohibitively high. Most patients may continue their primary VTE treatment regimen upon transition to secondary prevention at usual therapeutic doses for those on LMWH, VKAs (target INR 2.5, range 2.0–3.0), dabigatran, and edoxaban. Apixaban and rivaroxaban are approved for secondary VTE prevention at lower doses. Aspirin has some efficacy in mitigating VTE recurrence but is inferior to therapeutic anticoagulation (about 30% vs 80%–90% risk reduction).[83,84] It is a reasonable option in patients who refuse extended anticoagulation after the completion of the primary treatment phase if there is no contraindication to aspirin use. Extended anticoagulation should be avoided in patients with low VTE recurrence risk, such as women in whom VTE occurred while on oral contraceptives.

Consider the role of low-dose direct-acting oral anticoagulants. Extended therapy with low-dose DOAC (apixaban 2.5 mg twice daily or rivaroxaban 10 mg daily) decrease VTE recurrence with bleeding risks comparable to aspirin.[83] In patients where clinical equipoise exists (moderate risk of recurrent VTE and moderate bleeding risk), low-dose DOACs present a favorable net clinical benefit given their lower bleeding complications with extended therapy.[85] The efficacy of low-dose DOACs for secondary VTE prevention in high-recurrence risk patients (eg, active cancer) has not evaluated.[81]

DISCLOSURE

G.D. Barnes – consulting fees from Pfizer, Bristol-Myers Squibb, Jansen, Boston Scientific, Abbott Vascular, Bayer.

REFERENCES

1. Tsao CW, Aday AW, Almarzooq ZI, et al. Heart Disease and Stroke Statistics-2022 Update: A Report From the American Heart Association. Circulation 2022; 145(8):e153–639.
2. Cohen AT, Agnelli G, Anderson FA, et al. Venous thromboembolism (VTE) in Europe. The number of VTE events and associated morbidity and mortality. Thromb Haemost 2007;98(4):756–64.
3. Lutsey PL, Zakai NA. Epidemiology and prevention of venous thromboembolism. Nat Rev Cardiol 2022;1–15. https://doi.org/10.1038/s41569-022-00787-6.
4. Zakai NA, McClure LA, Judd SE, et al. Racial and regional differences in venous thromboembolism in the United States in 3 cohorts. Circulation 2014;129(14): 1502–9.
5. Wendelboe AM, Raskob GE. Global Burden of Thrombosis: Epidemiologic Aspects. Circ Res 2016;118(9):1340–7.
6. James AH. Venous thromboembolism in pregnancy. Arterioscler Thromb Vasc Biol 2009;29(3):326–31.
7. RIETE Registry. Death within 30 days: venous thromboembolism. Available at: https://rieteregistry.com/graphics-interactives/dead-30-days/.. Accessed April, 2021.
8. Renner E, Barnes GD. Antithrombotic Management of Venous Thromboembolism: JACC Focus Seminar. J Am Coll Cardiol 2020;76(18):2142–54.
9. Heit JA. Epidemiology of venous thromboembolism. Nat Rev Cardiol 2015;12(8): 464–74.
10. Ageno W, Farjat A, Haas S, et al. Provoked versus unprovoked venous thromboembolism: Findings from GARFIELD-VTE. Res Pract Thromb Haemost 2021;5(2): 326–41.

11. Khan F, Rahman A, Carrier M, et al. Long term risk of symptomatic recurrent venous thromboembolism after discontinuation of anticoagulant treatment for first unprovoked venous thromboembolism event: systematic review and meta-analysis. Bmj 2019;366:l4363.

12. Stevens SM, Woller SC, Kreuziger LB, et al. Antithrombotic Therapy for VTE Disease: Second Update of the CHEST Guideline and Expert Panel Report. Chest 2021;160(6):e545–608.

13. Mazzolai L, Ageno W, Alatri A, et al. Second consensus document on diagnosis and management of acute deep vein thrombosis: updated document elaborated by the ESC Working Group on aorta and peripheral vascular diseases and the ESC Working Group on pulmonary circulation and right ventricular function. Eur J Prev Cardiol 2022;29(8):1248–63.

14. Kearon C, Ageno W, Cannegieter SC, et al. Categorization of patients as having provoked or unprovoked venous thromboembolism: guidance from the SSC of ISTH. J Thromb Haemost 2016;14(7):1480–3.

15. Iorio A, Kearon C, Filippucci E, et al. Risk of recurrence after a first episode of symptomatic venous thromboembolism provoked by a transient risk factor: a systematic review. Arch Intern Med 2010;170(19):1710–6.

16. Konstantinides SV, Meyer G, Becattini C, et al. 2019 ESC Guidelines for the diagnosis and management of acute pulmonary embolism developed in collaboration with the European Respiratory Society (ERS): The Task Force for the diagnosis and management of acute pulmonary embolism of the European Society of Cardiology (ESC). Eur Respir J 2019;54(3). https://doi.org/10.1183/13993003.01647-2019.

17. Prandoni P, Lensing AW, Piccioli A, et al. Recurrent venous thromboembolism and bleeding complications during anticoagulant treatment in patients with cancer and venous thrombosis. Blood 2002;100(10):3484–8.

18. de Winter MA, van Es N, Büller HR, et al. Prediction models for recurrence and bleeding in patients with venous thromboembolism: A systematic review and critical appraisal. Thromb Res 2021;199:85–96.

19. Astruc N, Ianotto JC, Metges JP, et al. External validation of the modified Ottawa score for risk stratification of recurrent cancer-associated thrombosis. Eur J Intern Med 2016;36:e11–2.

20. Louzada ML, Bose G, Cheung A, et al. Predicting Venous Thromboembolism Recurrence Risk in Patients with Cancer: A Validation Study. Blood 2012; 120(21):394.

21. Freund Y, Cachanado M, Aubry A, et al. Effect of the Pulmonary Embolism Rule-Out Criteria on Subsequent Thromboembolic Events Among Low-Risk Emergency Department Patients: The PROPER Randomized Clinical Trial. JAMA 2018;319(6):559–66.

22. Carrier M, Righini M, Djurabi RK, et al. VIDAS D-dimer in combination with clinical pre-test probability to rule out pulmonary embolism. A systematic review of management outcome studies. Thromb Haemost 2009;101(5):886–92.

23. Haas FJ, Schutgens RE, Biesma DH. An age-adapted approach for the use of D-dimers in the exclusion of deep venous thrombosis. Am J Hematol 2009; 84(8):488–91.

24. Righini M, Van Es J, Den Exter PL, et al. Age-adjusted D-dimer cutoff levels to rule out pulmonary embolism: the ADJUST-PE study. JAMA 2014;311(11):1117–24.

25. Konstantinides SV, Meyer G, Becattini C, et al. 2019 ESC Guidelines for the diagnosis and management of acute pulmonary embolism developed in collaboration with the European Respiratory Society (ERS). Eur Heart J 2020;41(4):543–603.

26. Barnes GD, Muzikansky A, Cameron S, et al. Comparison of 4 Acute Pulmonary Embolism Mortality Risk Scores in Patients Evaluated by Pulmonary Embolism Response Teams. JAMA Netw Open 2020;3(8):e2010779.

27. Lyman GH, Carrier M, Ay C, et al. American Society of Hematology 2021 guidelines for management of venous thromboembolism: prevention and treatment in patients with cancer. Blood Adv 2021;5(4):927–74.

28. Delluc A, Antic D, Lecumberri R, et al. Occult cancer screening in patients with venous thromboembolism: guidance from the SSC of the ISTH. J Thromb Haemost 2017;15(10):2076–9.

29. McCormack T, Harrisingh MC, Horner D, et al. Venous thromboembolism in adults: summary of updated NICE guidance on diagnosis, management, and thrombophilia testing. Bmj 2020;369:m1565.

30. Favaloro EJ, McDonald D, Lippi G. Laboratory investigation of thrombophilia: the good, the bad, and the ugly. Semin Thromb Hemost 2009;35(7):695–710.

31. Dziadosz M, Baxi LV. Global prevalence of prothrombin gene mutation G20210A and implications in women's health: a systematic review. Blood Coagul Fibrinolysis 2016;27(5):481–9.

32. Weitz JI, Middeldorp S, Geerts W, et al. Thrombophilia and new anticoagulant drugs. Hematology Am Soc Hematol Educ Program 2004;424–38.

33. Middeldorp S, van Hylckama Vlieg A. Does thrombophilia testing help in the clinical management of patients? Br J Haematol 2008;143(3):321–35.

34. Van Cott EM, Khor B, Zehnder JL. Factor V Leiden. Am J Hematol 2016; 91(1):46–9.

35. Hooper WC, Dilley A, Ribeiro MJ, et al. A racial difference in the prevalence of the Arg506->Gln mutation. Thromb Res 1996;81(5):577–81.

36. Svensson PJ, Dahlbäck B. Resistance to activated protein C as a basis for venous thrombosis. N Engl J Med 1994;330(8):517–22.

37. Koster T, Rosendaal FR, de Ronde H, et al. Venous thrombosis due to poor anticoagulant response to activated protein C: Leiden Thrombophilia Study. Lancet 1993;342(8886–8887):1503–6.

38. Simone B, De Stefano V, Leoncini E, et al. Risk of venous thromboembolism associated with single and combined effects of Factor V Leiden, Prothrombin 20210A and Methylenetethraydrofolate reductase C677T: a meta-analysis involving over 11,000 cases and 21,000 controls. Eur J Epidemiol 2013;28(8):621–47.

39. Poort SR, Rosendaal FR, Reitsma PH, et al. A common genetic variation in the 3'-untranslated region of the prothrombin gene is associated with elevated plasma prothrombin levels and an increase in venous thrombosis. Blood 1996;88(10):3698–703.

40. Meyer MR, Witt DM, Delate T, et al. Thrombophilia testing patterns amongst patients with acute venous thromboembolism. Thromb Res 2015;136(6):1160–4.

41. Cooper PC, Goodeve AC, Beauchamp NJ. Quality in molecular biology testing for inherited thrombophilia disorders. Semin Thromb Hemost 2012;38(6):600–12.

42. Clouse LH, Comp PC. The regulation of hemostasis: the protein C system. N Engl J Med 1986;314(20):1298–304.

43. Koster T, Rosendaal FR, Briët E, et al. Protein C deficiency in a controlled series of unselected outpatients: an infrequent but clear risk factor for venous thrombosis (Leiden Thrombophilia Study). Blood 1995;85(10):2756–61.

44. Lipe B, Ornstein DL. Deficiencies of natural anticoagulants, protein C, protein S, and antithrombin. Circulation 2011;124(14):e365–8.

45. Cooper PC, Hill M, Maclean RM. The phenotypic and genetic assessment of protein C deficiency. Int J Lab Hematol 2012;34(4):336–46.

46. Nizzi FA Jr, Kaplan HS. Protein C and S deficiency. Semin Thromb Hemost 1999; 25(3):265–72.
47. Marciniak E, Wilson HD, Marlar RA. Neonatal purpura fulminans: a genetic disorder related to the absence of protein C in blood. Blood 1985;65(1):15–20.
48. Cooper PC, Pavlova A, Moore GW, et al. Recommendations for clinical laboratory testing for protein C deficiency, for the subcommittee on plasma coagulation inhibitors of the ISTH. J Thromb Haemost 2020;18(2):271–7.
49. Dahlbäck B. The tale of protein S and C4b-binding protein, a story of affection. Thromb Haemost 2007;98(1):90–6.
50. Castoldi E, Hackeng TM. Regulation of coagulation by protein S. Curr Opin Hematol 2008;15(5):529–36.
51. Hackeng TM, Seré KM, Tans G, et al. Protein S stimulates inhibition of the tissue factor pathway by tissue factor pathway inhibitor. Proc Natl Acad Sci U S A 2006; 103(9):3106–11.
52. García de Frutos P, Fuentes-Prior P, Hurtado B, et al. Molecular basis of protein S deficiency. Thromb Haemost 2007;98(3):543–56.
53. Beauchamp NJ, Dykes AC, Parikh N. Campbell Tait R, Daly ME. The prevalence of, and molecular defects underlying, inherited protein S deficiency in the general population. Br J Haematol 2004;125(5):647–54.
54. Inherited thrombophilia. memorandum from a joint WHO/International Society on Thrombosis and Haemostasis meeting. Bull World Health Organ 1997;75(3): 177–89.
55. Marlar RA, Gausman JN. Protein S abnormalities: a diagnostic nightmare. Am J Hematol 2011;86(5):418–21.
56. Patnaik MM, Moll S. Inherited antithrombin deficiency: a review. Haemophilia 2008;14(6):1229–39.
57. De Stefano V, Finazzi G, Mannucci PM. Inherited thrombophilia: pathogenesis, clinical syndromes, and management. Blood 1996;87(9):3531–44.
58. Khor B, Van Cott EM. Laboratory tests for antithrombin deficiency. Am J Hematol 2010;85(12):947–50.
59. Durcan L, Petri M. Chapter 2-Epidemiology of the Antiphospholipid Syndrome. In: Cervera R, Espinosa G, Khamashta M, editors. Handbook of systemic autoimmune diseases. Elsevier; 2017. p. 17–30.
60. Petri M. Epidemiology of the antiphospholipid antibody syndrome. J Autoimmun 2000;15(2):145–51.
61. Hughes GR. Thrombosis, abortion, cerebral disease, and the lupus anticoagulant. Br Med J 1983;287(6399):1088–9.
62. Miyakis S, Lockshin MD, Atsumi T, et al. International consensus statement on an update of the classification criteria for definite antiphospholipid syndrome (APS). J Thromb Haemost 2006;4(2):295–306.
63. Cohen H, Efthymiou M, Devreese KMJ. Monitoring of anticoagulation in thrombotic antiphospholipid syndrome. J Thromb Haemost 2021;19(4):892–908.
64. Ho WK, Hankey GJ, Quinlan DJ, et al. Risk of recurrent venous thromboembolism in patients with common thrombophilia: a systematic review. Arch Intern Med 2006;166(7):729–36.
65. Kearon C, Akl EA, Comerota AJ, et al. Antithrombotic therapy for VTE disease: Antithrombotic Therapy and Prevention of Thrombosis, 9th ed: American College of Chest Physicians Evidence-Based Clinical Practice Guidelines. Chest 2012; 141(2 Suppl):e419S–96S.

66. Marchetti M, Pistorio A, Barosi G. Extended anticoagulation for prevention of recurrent venous thromboembolism in carriers of factor V Leiden–cost-effectiveness analysis. Thromb Haemost 2000;84(5):752–7.

67. Vink R, Kraaijenhagen RA, Levi M, et al. Individualized duration of oral anticoagulant therapy for deep vein thrombosis based on a decision model. J Thromb Haemost 2003;1(12):2523–30.

68. Couturaud F, Leroyer C, Tromeur C, et al. Factors that predict thrombosis in relatives of patients with venous thromboembolism. Blood 2014;124(13):2124–30.

69. Arachchillage DJ, Mackillop L, Chandratheva A, et al. Thrombophilia testing: A British Society for Haematology guideline. Br J Haematol 2022;198(3):443–58.

70. Hellmann EA, Leslie ND, Moll S. Knowledge and educational needs of individuals with the factor V Leiden mutation. J Thromb Haemost 2003;1(11):2335–9.

71. Connors JM. Thrombophilia Testing and Venous Thrombosis. N Engl J Med 2017;377(12):1177–87.

72. Deloughery TG, Hunt BJ, Barnes GD, et al. A call to action: MTHFR polymorphisms should not be a part of inherited thrombophilia testing. Res Pract Thromb Haemost 2022;6(4):e12739.

73. Lonn E, Yusuf S, Arnold MJ, et al. Homocysteine lowering with folic acid and B vitamins in vascular disease. N Engl J Med 2006;354(15):1567–77.

74. Kearon C. A conceptual framework for two phases of anticoagulant treatment of venous thromboembolism. J Thromb Haemost 2012;10(4):507–11.

75. Boutitie F, Pinede L, Schulman S, et al. Influence of preceding length of anticoagulant treatment and initial presentation of venous thromboembolism on risk of recurrence after stopping treatment: analysis of individual participants' data from seven trials. Bmj 2011;342:d3036.

76. Ageno W, Donadini M. Breadth of complications of long-term oral anticoagulant care. Hematology Am Soc Hematol Educ Program 2018;2018(1):432–8.

77. Carrier M, Le Gal G, Wells PS, et al. Systematic review: case-fatality rates of recurrent venous thromboembolism and major bleeding events among patients treated for venous thromboembolism. Ann Intern Med 2010;152(9):578–89.

78. Kakkos SK, Kirkilesis GI, Tsolakis IA. 's Choice - efficacy and safety of the new oral anticoagulants dabigatran, rivaroxaban, apixaban, and edoxaban in the treatment and secondary prevention of venous thromboembolism: a systematic review and meta-analysis of phase III trials. Eur J Vasc Endovasc Surg 2014;48(5):565–75.

79. Mai V, Bertoletti L, Cucherat M, et al. Extended anticoagulation for the secondary prevention of venous thromboembolic events: An updated network meta-analysis. PLoS One 2019;14(4):e0214134.

80. Li A, Garcia DA, Lyman GH, et al. Direct oral anticoagulant (DOAC) versus low-molecular-weight heparin (LMWH) for treatment of cancer associated thrombosis (CAT): A systematic review and meta-analysis. Thromb Res 2019;173:158–63.

81. Ortel TL, Neumann I, Ageno W, et al. American Society of Hematology 2020 guidelines for management of venous thromboembolism: treatment of deep vein thrombosis and pulmonary embolism. Blood Adv 2020;4(19):4693–738.

82. Khan F, Tritschler T, Kimpton M, et al. Long-Term Risk for Major Bleeding During Extended Oral Anticoagulant Therapy for First Unprovoked Venous Thromboembolism : A Systematic Review and Meta-analysis. Ann Intern Med 2021;174(10):1420–9.

83. Weitz JI, Lensing AWA, Prins MH, et al. Rivaroxaban or Aspirin for Extended Treatment of Venous Thromboembolism. N Engl J Med 2017;376(13):1211–22.

84. Becattini C, Agnelli G, Schenone A, et al. Aspirin for preventing the recurrence of venous thromboembolism. N Engl J Med 2012;366(21):1959–67.
85. Serhal M, Barnes GD. Venous thromboembolism: A clinician update. Vasc Med 2019;24(2):122–31.
86. Tai SMM, Buddhdev P, Baskaradas A, et al. Venous thromboembolism in the trauma patient. Orthopaedics and Trauma 2013;27(6):379–92.
87. Lee Y, Jehangir Q, Li P, et al. Venous thromboembolism in COVID-19 patients and prediction model: a multicenter cohort study. BMC Infect Dis 2022;22(1):462.
88. Mahajan A, Brunson A, White R, et al. The Epidemiology of Cancer-Associated Venous Thromboembolism: An Update. Semin Thromb Hemost 2019;45(4):321–5.
89. Kearon C, Iorio A, Palareti G. Risk of recurrent venous thromboembolism after stopping treatment in cohort studies: recommendation for acceptable rates and standardized reporting. J Thromb Haemost 2010;8(10):2313–5.
90. Franco Moreno AI, García Navarro MJ, Ortiz Sánchez J, et al. A risk score for prediction of recurrence in patients with unprovoked venous thromboembolism (DAMOVES). Eur J Intern Med 2016;29:59–64.
91. Timp JF, Braekkan SK, Lijfering WM, et al. Correction: Prediction of recurrent venous thrombosis in all patients with a first venous thrombotic event: The Leiden Thrombosis Recurrence Risk Prediction model (L-TRRiP). PLoS Med 2021;18(4): e1003612.
92. Nendaz M, Spirk D, Kucher N, et al. Multicentre validation of the Geneva Risk Score for hospitalised medical patients at risk of venous thromboembolism. Explicit ASsessment of Thromboembolic RIsk and Prophylaxis for Medical PA-Tients in SwitzErland (ESTIMATE). Thromb Haemost 2014;111(3):531–8.
93. Wells PS, Anderson DR, Bormanis J, et al. Value of assessment of pretest probability of deep-vein thrombosis in clinical management. Lancet 1997;350(9094): 1795–8.

Venous Thromboembolism
The Need for Transitions of Care

Anthony Joseph Macchiavelli, MD

KEYWORDS

- Venous thromboembolism • Inferior vena cava filters • SHM FAST

KEY POINTS

- Patients transitioning from the hospital setting with VTE are vulnerable due to multiple factors inherent in current care models.
- The concern over adverse drug events associated with anticoagulation potentially leading to re-hospitalization and harm deserves special attention.
- There are new and innovative programs, such as SHM FAST, that specifically target this patient population.

INTRODUCTION

The Centers for Disease Control and Prevention estimates that approximately 900,000 patients are diagnosed with venous thromboembolism (VTE) annually in the United States leading to approximately 548,000 hospitalizations and 100,000 deaths.[1] Approximately 274 people die daily in the United States from VTE. The numbers are staggering with 1 person dying every 5 minutes! There are more deaths annually in the United States from VTE than breast cancer (41,000), AIDS (16,000), and motor vehicle accidents (32,000) combined![1] VTE is recognized as a leading cause of preventable hospital deaths and a leading cause of maternal deaths. The health care costs associated with VTE in the United States are estimated at $7-10 billion.[2] What is most notable is that VTE is preventable. Additionally, the harm associated with the treatment of VTE is preventable. However, problems surface when patients with VTE transition from one level of care to another. For instance, the patient discharged from the hospital is at risk of potential harm from discontinuity of care. This problem can also be seen with transitions in patients with other diagnoses, but patients with VTE are at increased risk for adverse drug events and re-admissions.

FACTORS IMPACTING TRANSITIONS OF CARE

When patients transition from the hospital to other settings, several challenges arise. There is a potential risk of losing important information regarding patient care. Harm

Division Vascular Medicine, Jefferson Vascular Center, Sidney Kimmel Medical College, 111 South 11th Street, 6210 Gibbon, Philadelphia, PA 19107, USA
E-mail address: Anthony.Macchiavelli@jefferson.edu

Med Clin N Am 107 (2023) 883–894
https://doi.org/10.1016/j.mcna.2023.05.001
0025-7125/23/© 2023 Elsevier Inc. All rights reserved.

can arise as the patient leaves the hospital setting without appropriate handoff of key elements such as hospital course, medication changes, and aftercare plan. Many current hospital systems create a discontinuity of care between sending and receiving providers with a potential for harm. In some hospital settings, primary care providers have limited involvement in the care of their patients with whom they have developed long-term relationships. Often hospital care is provided by the hospital-based team led by a Hospitalist, an ED Provider, and or an Intensivist. The primary care provider may not be involved at all during the hospitalization other than through telephone communications with the hospital treatment team. Handoffs between sending and receiving providers should occur at key transition points, such as admission or discharge from a facility or unit, and this creates a potential for significant communication breakdown. Sometimes, there is no handoff, potentially worsening the situation.[3] Also, within health care settings such as hospitals, communication can be fragmented among providers as a patient transition from one unit to another, commonly having a new set of providers.

This transition of care at discharge is further complicated by the vulnerable patient who may not fully understand everything explained and is presented with an overwhelming amount of information at discharge. The volume of information presented can be staggering for a patient. The patient discharge instructions packet includes a large volume of information that is aimed at providing comprehensive directions, but it often fails at effectively communicating key elements such as aftercare plans and medication changes. The discharge instructions may not have been written in simple-to-understand language. Often instructions contain medical jargon that may be difficult for a non-medical person to understand. The discharge instructions may not be in the spoken language of the patient. Moreover, it is common for a patient to hear only part of the information during an overwhelming time, such as discharge from the hospital. Even highly functioning patients may not understand everything in their after-care plan. However, there are strategies to help bridge this problem. The term health literacy is used to assess a patient's understanding of key elements such as diagnosis, aftercare plan, and medication changes. Having the patient repeat back these key elements to better assess their level of understanding and make necessary adjustments can be an effective approach. This approach is called "Teach Back."[4,5] When patients have difficulty with "Teach Back," using a family member or proxy may help ensure a seamless transition.

The discontinuity between the hospital-based care team and the primary care team may lead to failed handoffs with potential adverse consequences. Patients often have test results pending at the time of discharge that require follow-up. The receiving providers may be unaware that there are results that require further action.[6] Discharge summaries afford a method of redundancy that allows receiving providers an overview of their patient's hospitalization, but often these summaries are missing key information that may adversely impact patient care.[7,8] Of course, provider-to-provider direct communication is optimal, allowing the receiving provider the opportunity to ask questions. Unfortunately, this type of communication is highly variable and often does not occur.

Another key element to a safe transition is the follow up of the patient with the aftercare provider. Often patients are lost to follow up, or they follow up outside of a window of time for safe care. In some cases, patients are discharged to another care facility such as acute rehabilitation, skilled nursing facility, long-term acute care hospital (LTACH) or long-term care facility. When this type of transition occurs an additional care team may become involved with the potential loss of information and loss of continuity. At every step of the transition there is a risk for error, and the more steps, the greater risk. This problem can also be seen with medications leading to potential harm.

Medication reconciliation is an important process during transitions verifying patient's medications and noting medications that have been started or discontinued. The performance of medication reconciliation is an ongoing process at key points of transition. The complexity of medication treatments has grown and there are medications, such as anticoagulants that can have dire consequences if taken incorrectly. Additionally, it is a time for the clinician to review how patients take their medications. Confusion about dosing schedules and self-administration can be detected by the clinician during this evaluation. Unfortunately, if an appropriate medication reconciliation does not occur and unnecessary redundancies, expired or incorrect dosages, or the wrong medications are not corrected, then the patient is at risk for harm.

Complicating the issue of safe transitions is the reduction in the length of stay of a patient during hospitalization. Some patients are discharged with VTE from the emergency department. In some instances, patients with VTE are treated completely in the outpatient setting.

RISK WITH ANTICOAGULANTS AND VENOUS THROMBOEMBOLISM

In 2012 Budnitz and colleagues[9] estimated that the rates of emergency hospitalizations for adverse drug events in older adults from 2007 to 2009 were highest for warfarin, accounting for 20 hospitalizations per 10,000 outpatient visits. It should be noted that warfarin was the only anticoagulant studied. Antiplatelet medications were also associated with adverse drug events leading to re-hospitalization in this study. Since this study, we have seen the emergence of direct oral anticoagulants (DOACs) with indications for VTE and atrial fibrillation. There are currently 4 FDA-approved DOACs in the US for the treatment of VTE: Apixaban, Dabigatran, Edoxaban, and Rivaroxaban (**Table 1**). Due to the efficacy and safety of these agents, the current guidelines recommend the use of apixaban, dabigatran, edoxaban or rivaroxaban in the treatment of VTE over vitamin K antagonists such as warfarin.[10,11] In patients with cancer-associated VTE, apixaban, edoxaban, or rivaroxaban are recommended over low molecular weight heparin.[10] However, if a patient has confirmed antiphospholipid syndrome, a vitamin K antagonist is recommended over the DOACs.[10] Additionally, patients with low-risk DVT and PE are recommended to have outpatient treatment rather than inpatient treatment for VTE.[10,11] So how is the risk for patients with VTE assessed?

Patients at risk for mortality from PE can be assessed using prognostic models such as the Pulmonary Embolism Severity Index (PESI)[12] or a simplified PESI (sPESI),[13] HESTIA, or BOVA scores. The PESI and sPESI score have been validated with the best results for patients at low risk for 30-day mortality.[11] The PESI score assigns points and evaluates variables such as age, male gender, history of cancer, heart failure, chronic lung disease, pulse $\geq$ 110/min, systolic blood pressure <100 mm Hg, respiratory rate $\geq$ 30/min, temperature < 36o Celsius, altered mental status, and arterial oxygen < 90%. Class I (<66 points) and Class II (66 to 85 points) are low risk for 30-day mortality. Class III (86 to 105 points), Class IV (106 to 125 points), and Class V (>125 points) are high risk. But the calculation can be cumbersome. Therefore, the sPESI was developed to facilitate clinicians making calculations for the risk of death from PE. The sPESI score assigns 1 point for age > 80 years, history of cancer, chronic cardiopulmonary disease, pulse $\geq$ 110/min, systolic blood pressure < 100 mm Hg, and arterial oxygen saturation < 90%. Low-risk patients have an sPESI score of 0; high-risk patients have an sPESI score $\geq$ 1.

The Hestia Score also evaluates patients at low risk who may be eligible for outpatient management.[14] This score evaluates hemodynamic instability, thrombolysis or

Table 1
Direct oral anticoagulants used in the treatment of acute VTE

DOAC	Mechanism	Half-Life	Peak Onset	Parenteral Lead in Required?	Dosing
Apixaban	Factor Xa inhibitor	11.5 h	1.5–3.3 h	No	10 mg twice daily for 7 days, then 5 mg twice daily
Dabigatran	Direct thrombin inhibitor	12–14 h	2 h	Yes[a]	150 mg twice daily
Edoxaban	Factor Xa inhibitor	10–14 h	1.5 h	Yes[a]	60 mg daily
Rivaroxaban	Factor Xa inhibitor	5–9 h	2–4 h	No	15 mg twice daily for 21 days then 20 mg daily

[a] After 5 days can transition to oral.
Modified from Merli G, Hiestand B, Amin A, et al. Balancing Anti-thrombotic Efficacy and Bleeding Risk in the Contemporary Management of Venous Thromboembolism. Curr Emerg Hosp Med Rep; 07 April 2015: 3 89-99.

embolectomy needed, active bleeding or high risk for bleeding, >24 hours on supplemental oxygen to maintain a SaO2 > 90%, PE diagnosed on anticoagulation, severe pain needing intravenous pain medication required > 24 hours, medical or social reason for admission, creatinine clearance < 30 mL/min by Cockcroft-Gault formula, severe liver impairment, pregnant, or history of heparin-induced thrombocytopenia. If 1 or more is present, the patient is not recommended for outpatient management (**Table 2**).

Finally, the BOVA score aims to identify patients with intermediate-risk PE.[15] This score assigns 2 points each for SBP 90-100 mm Hg, elevated cardiac troponin, and RV dysfunction on echocardiogram or CT scan. It assigns 1 point for a heart rate > 110 beats per minute. A score of 0-2 is Stage I and considered low risk with PE-related complications at 4.4% and PE-related mortality at 3.1%. A score of 3-4 is Stage II and is intermediate risk, with PE complications at 18% and PE-related mortality at 6.8%. A score >4 is Stage III and high risk with PE complications at 42% and PE-related mortality at 10% (**Fig. 1**).

The use of these scores can help guide clinicians caring for patients with PE with risk stratification and site of care. The scores also highlight the vulnerability of patients with VTE and the risk of mortality associated with PE.

CENTER FOR MEDICARE AND MEDICAID SERVICES MEASURES TO PREVENT READMISSIONS FOCUS ON CREATING SAFE TRANSITIONS

The Joint Commission recognized the vulnerability of patients receiving anticoagulation and developed the National Patient Safety Goal for anticoagulant therapy.[16] The aim of this effort is stated later in discussion:

Table 2 The hestia score		
Is the patient hemodynamically unstable?[a]	Yes	No
Is thrombolysis or embolectomy necessary?	Yes	No
Active bleeding or hign risk of bleeding[b]	Yes	No
More than 24 h of oxygen supply to maintain oxygen saturation > 90%?	Yes	No
Is pulmonary embolism diagnosed during anticoagulant treatment?	Yes	No
Severa pain needing intravenous pain medication for mote than 24 h	Yes	No
Medical or social reason for treatment in the hospital for more than 24 h (infection, malignancy, no support system)?	Yes	No
Does the ptient ghave a creatinine clearance of < 30 mL min^{-1}?[c]	Yes	No
Does the patient have severe liver impairment?[d]	Yes	No
Is the patient pregnant	Yes	No
Does the patient have a documented history of heparin-induced thrombocytoprnia?	Yes	No
If the answer to one of the questions is 'yes', the patient cannot be teeated at home in the Hestia Study		

[a] Include the following criteria, but leave these to the discretion of the investigator: systolic blood pressure < 100 mm Hg with heart rate > 100 beats min^{-1}; condition requiring admission to an intensive care unit.
[b] Gastrointestinal bledding in the preceding 14 days, recent stroke (< 4 weeks ago), recent operation (< 2 weeks ago), bleeding disorder or thrombocytopenia (platelet count < 75 × 109 L^{-1}), uncontrolled hypertension (systolic blood pressure > 180 mm Hg or diastolic blood pressure > 110 mm Hg).
[c] Calculated creatinine clearance according to the Cockroft-Gaukt formula.
[d] Left to the discretion of the physican.
Taken from Zondag W, Mos ICM, Creemers-Schild D, et al. Outpatient treatment in patients with acute pulmonary embolism: the Hestia study. J Thromb Haemost. 2011; 9(8):1500-1507.

The 8P Screening Tool
Identifying Your Patient's Risk for Adverse Events After Discharge

The 8Ps (Check all that apply.)	Risk Specific Intervention	Signature of individual responsible for insuring intervention administered
Problems with medications (polypharmacy – i.e. ≥10 routine meds – or high risk medication including: insulin, anticoagulants, oral hypoglycemic agents, dual antiplatelet therapy, digoxin, or narcotics) ☐	☐ Medication specific education using Teach Back provided to patient and caregiver ☐ Monitoring plan developed and communicated to patient and aftercare providers, where relevant (e.g. warfarin, digoxin and insulin) ☐ Specific strategies for managing adverse drug events reviewed with patient/caregiver ☐ Elimination of unnecessary medications ☐ Simplification of medication scheduling to improve adherence ☐ Follow-up phone call at 72 h to assess adherence and complications	
Psychological (depression screen positive or history of depression diagnosis) ☐	☐ Assessment of need for psychiatric care if not in place ☐ Communication with primary care provider, highlighting this issue if new ☐ Involvement/awareness of support network insured	
Principal diagnosis (cancer, stroke, DM, COPD, heart failure) ☐	☐ Review of national discharge guidelines, where available ☐ Disease specific education using Teach Back with patient/caregiver ☐ Action plan reviewed with patient/caregivers regarding what to do and who to contact in the event of worsening or new symptoms ☐ Discuss goals of care and chronic illness model discussed with patient/caregiver	
Physical limitations (deconditioning, frailty, malnutrition or other physical limitations that impair their ability to participate in their care) ☐	☐ Engage family/caregivers to ensure ability to assist with post-discharge care assistance ☐ Assessment of home services to address limitations and care needs ☐ Follow-up phone call at 72 h to assess ability to adhere to the care plan with services and support in place.	
Poor health literacy (inability to do Teach Back) ☐	☐ Committed caregiver involved in planning/administration of all discharge planning and general and risk specific interventions ☐ Post-hospital care plan education using Teach Back provided to patient and caregiver ☐ Link to community resources for additional patient/caregiver support ☐ Follow-up phone call at 72 h to assess adherence and complications	
Patient support (social isolation, absence of support to assist with care, as well as insufficient or absent connection with primary care) ☐	☐ Follow-up phone call at 72 h to assess condition, adherence and complications ☐ Follow-up appointment with appropriate medical provider within 7 d after hospitalization ☐ Involvement of home care providers of services with clear communications of discharge plan to those providers ☐ Engage a transition coach	
Prior hospitalization (non-elective; in last 6 months) ☐	☐ Review reasons for re-hospitalization in context of prior hospitalization ☐ Follow-up phone call at 72 h to assess condition, adherence and complications ☐ Follow-up appointment with medical provider within 7 d of hospital discharge ☐ Engage a transition coach	
Palliative care (Would you be surprised if this patient died in the next year? Does this patient have an advanced or progressive serious illness? "No" to 1st or "Yes" to 2nd = positive screen) ☐	☐ Assess need for palliative care services ☐ Identify goals of care and therapeutic options ☐ Communicate prognosis with patient/family/caregiver ☐ Assess and address concerning symptoms ☐ Identify services or benefits available to patients based on advanced disease status ☐ Discuss with patient/caregiver role of palliative care services and the benefits and services available to the patient	

Fig. 1. The BOOST 8Ps. (*Taken from* Coffey C, Greenwald J, Budnitz T, et al. Project BOOST Implementation Guide, second edition. 2013; Appendix K p.136.)

"NPSG.03.05.01: Reduce the likelihood of patient harm associated with the use of anticoagulant therapy."

The focus of this safety goal is to minimize the risk to the patient taking anticoagulants by ensuring appropriate evidence-based protocols are implemented, including the monitoring of drug-to-drug interactions, drug to food interactions, INR, renal and/or liver function when appropriate. Additionally, monitoring and reporting of adverse drug events, strategies for patient education, and strategies for managing the bleeding patient are discussed.[16]

READMISSION RISK STRATIFICATION AT TRANSITION

Risk assessment evaluation using screening tools has been used to identify patients during transitions of care who are at high risk for readmissions. The Society of Hospital Medicine developed a program called Project BOOST (Better Outcomes by Optimizing Safe Transitions) to address this challenge. BOOST identifies 8 problem areas and provides key interventions to avoid adverse events for patients discharged from the hospital. They are known as the "8Ps" (see **Fig. 1**). "Problems with Medications" is one of the 8Ps that identifies two areas: (1) polypharmacy with patients receiving 10 or more routine medications and (2) High-risk medications such as anticoagulants, dual antiplatelet therapy, diabetic medications, and narcotics as a potential risk for adverse events.[5] Specific interventions include medication education using "Teach Back," a monitoring plan developed and communicated to the patient and aftercare providers, strategies to manage adverse drug events, elimination of unnecessary medications, simplified scheduling and follow up phone call at 72 hours to better assess adherence and complications.[5] A limitation of the 8Ps for patients with VTE can be seen in the category "Principle Diagnosis." This category includes cancer, stroke, diabetes, COPD, and heart failure, but does not specifically address VTE.[5] This risk assessment model does consider other areas such as "Poor Health Literacy," defined as inability to do teach back, and "Physical Limitations" as key problems at transition. There is no score in this model since its focus addresses specific vulnerabilities during transition and places action steps to create better outcomes.

Other readmission risk assessment strategies can be found in the HOSPITAL score and the LACE index. The HOSPITAL score (**Table 3**) is a validated score and considers the variables hemoglobin, discharge from the oncology service, sodium, procedure during the hospitalization, index type admission as elective or non-elective and hospital length of stay $\geq$ 5 days. Patients with a HOSPITAL score of 7 or greater are at risk for readmission to the hospital.[17] However, this score does not specifically address anticoagulation or VTE.

Finally, the LACE index[18] considers the length of stay, patient acuity on admission, and comorbid illness as measured using the Charlson index and Emergency Department utilization in the last 6 months. The Charlson index does mention peripheral vascular disease but does not specifically mention VTE.[19]

With the challenges and limitations of risk stratification, identifying patients at risk during transitions with venous thromboembolism and the vulnerability of patients with VTE, a different strategy must be undertaken for this disease-specific transition need. Other solutions have surfaced to reduce harm.

Harm Reduction Strategies

With more complex management and a growing number of anticoagulants and indications, the role of the Pharmacist in transitions has had a positive impact on

Table 3
The HOSPITAL score

Attribute	Points
Low hemoglobin level at discharge (<12 g/dL)	1
Discharge from an oncology service	2
Low sodium level at discharge (<135 mEq/L)	1
Procedure during hospital stay (any ICD-9-CM coded procedure)	1
Index admission type: nonelective	1
Number of hospital admissions during the previous year	
0	0
1–5	2
>5	5
Length of stay $\geq$ 5 days	2

Readmission Risk	Score
Low	0–4
Intermediate	5–6
High	$\geq$ 7

Modified from Donzé J, Aujesky D, Williams D, Schnipper JL. Potentially Avoidable 30-Day Hospital Readmissions in Medical Patients: Derivation and Validation of a Prediction Model. JAMA Intern Med. 2013; 173(8):632–638.

bridging the care gap by improving patient understanding and appropriate use of anticoagulants but has not significantly reduced bleeding or 30-readmissions.[20,21] One possible explanation surfaced from a study of patients from Project RED (Re-Engineered Discharge),[22] where 401 patients were identified, 277 received a pharmacist call and 124 could not be contacted. Patients who could not be contacted were more likely to be readmitted or visit the emergency department. The importance of the connection with the patient at transition or discharge and the connection between the sending provider team and the receiving team is paramount to a safe transition. However, despite all efforts for appropriate management, it can be expected that a subset of patients will fail in transitions and require more frequent health care contact than others. For instance, reconciliation with insurers for approval for a specific medication may not occur correctly or timely at discharge. Patients may present to the pharmacy and receive a bill for hundreds of dollars because the insurer did not approve the medication or has another medication on the formulary. Additionally, the patient who is discharged after normal business hours or on weekends may require special arrangements. One countermeasure includes delivering the medication to the patient's bed prior to discharge. The strategy ensures that the patient has the medications in hand when they are discharged from the hospital. It eliminates a potential extra step when treatment delays could occur and potentially contribute to harm. Pharmaceutical companies have simplified the process with payment vouchers and samples. Another innovation from pharmaceutical companies is a blister pack for the first 30 days of treatment for newly diagnosed venous thromboembolism. This pack helps bridge a medication error that may occur as the patient transitions from the hospital or the Emergency Department. DOACs such as edoxaban and dabigatran require a parenteral lead in therapy for approximately 5 days prior to starting the DOAC. This additional step requires parenteral administration with a medication such as heparin infusion targeting a therapeutic aPTT or a low molecular weight heparin administered subcutaneously. An advantage of low molecular weight heparin is that it may be administered in the outpatient setting and potentially shortens hospital length of stay. The disadvantage is the required training of the patient or a proxy on the injection of the low molecular weight heparin. It is usually easier to take a pill than to self-inject for patients. The situation is more complicated if the patient is managed with warfarin, usually requiring the titration of an INR to a therapeutic level of 2 – 3. This approach may require bridging with a parenteral anticoagulant such as heparin or a low molecular weight heparin. The additional blood draws required during titration and subsequent periodic monitoring complicate the management strategy and create opportunities for treatment failure. Close monitoring by a care team such as an anticoagulation clinic can reduce harm in this situation. The time in therapeutic range of INR for warfarin monitoring is a significant metric for high-quality anticoagulation management. Dedicated teams, such as anticoagulation clinics, may be more successful than traditional office-based monitoring since care is focused on the complexity of anticoagulation management. Nevertheless, even in the best-controlled anticoagulation studies with DOACs, the time in the therapeutic range falls short of perfect. In some of the best-controlled studies, the time in the therapeutic range was at best 63.5%.[23] This implies that the patient was either under-anticoagulated and at risk of clotting or over-anticoagulated and at greater risk of bleeding. The DOACs have stopped the complexity of monitoring INRs, but renal function, liver function, blood count, and drug-to-drug interaction still require evaluation. Patients taking CYP3A4 Inducers and Inhibitors, and P-glycoprotein Inducers and Inhibitors may have strong interactions with the DOACs and may need to be avoided or closely monitored. Similarly, these drugs should not be used during pregnancy or during breastfeeding. Patients using nonsteroidal anti-inflammatory drugs (NSAIDS) are at increased risk for bleeding while taking anticoagulants and require education on alternate or safer therapies. These issues could be monitored in high-quality anticoagulation clinics.

Venous Thromboembolism and the Inferior Vena Cava Filters

Some patients diagnosed with VTE require the placement of an IVC filter. In most instances, the filter is only temporary and should be removed as early as possible. When patients are transitioning from the hospital setting after the placement of an IVC filter, the follow-up for removal of the filter should be communicated and, if possible, scheduled. Indwelling retrievable filters that are not removed increases the risk of harm.

SPECIFIC PROGRAMS AIMED AT CREATING SAFE TRANSITIONS: SOCIETY OF HOSPITAL MEDICINE FACILITATION OF ANTICOAGULATION FOR SAFER TRANSITIONS

Programs such as Project BOOST offer a powerful approach to creating a model for safe transitions, but a greater focus on patients transitioning from hospitals with VTE is necessary to address the complexities associated with this disease state and its treatment. A novel program that specifically addresses transitions of care for patients with VTE is the Society of Hospital Medicine Facilitation of Anticoagulation for Safer Transitions (SHM FAST) program.[24] This program originated as a quality improvement effort directed to help patients safely transition from the hospital with VTE. It is a mentored program that started at multiple sites across a mix of academic and community hospitals of varying sizes. The sites met monthly with mentors and assembled interdisciplinary teams consisting of a Lead Hospitalist, Lead Pharmacist, Lead Nurse, Lead Primary Care Provider, and Lead Information Technology Specialist. Additional members were added based on individual site needs. The goal of this quality improvement program was for sites to address the needs of patients diagnosed with VTE transitioning from the hospital setting by creating a seamless process leveraging the assets within each institution. The targets were both process and outcome measures facilitating safe transitions. Patients were included in the program if there was a primary ICD-10 code for acute DVT or PE. Patients were excluded if they were not discharged on full anticoagulation, had chronic VTE or acute VTE that is not their primary diagnosis during hospitalization, refused treatment or follow-up care, or could not be transitioned to an ambulatory setting for safety reasons or social situations in which would prevent communication with the patient for follow up care (such as homeless with no phone or means to contact). The sites used evidence-based transition protocols incorporating either a standard or a comprehensive bundle. The standard bundle was used by most of the sites in this program. The components of the standard bundle are listed later in discussion.

- Perform a 2-day follow-up call.
- Perform enhanced medication reconciliation.
- Utilize the VTE order set.
- Employ a checklist for oral anticoagulation readiness.
- Utilize the checklist for DOAC appropriateness.
- Use a standardized discharge readiness checklist.
- Utilize standardized transition record.
- Hospitalist will directly communicate the plan of care to the next provider using a standardized script

The Comprehensive Bundle included all components of the standard bundle plus the following.

- Perform a face-to-face visit within 7 days post-discharge.
- Oversee patient care for 30 days post-discharge.
- Perform 30-day phone calls.

There were 3 phases to this process. The first phase was a baseline assessment and goal setting over a 3-month period to evaluate institutional assets and gaps in the transition process for patients with VTE. Process mapping was initiated during this phase aimed at understanding current processes at each institution. The focus was to develop attainable goals that were specific, measurable, achievable, relevant, and time-bound (SMART goals). Efforts were then mobilized to achieve those goals. Evaluating change that occurred throughout the process used the Plan-Do-Study-Act (PDSA) cycle. The second phase was an implementation phase over a 12-month period during which the plan was executed with adjustments made as needed. The final phase was a 3-month sustainability phase looking at the success of the efforts the team accomplished in the prior phases in creating the transitions and ensuring it was hard wired into the fabric of the institution.[24]

In this program, 1,995 patients were screened for eligibility and 1,322 were enrolled in the program. Results provide a signal in the right direction for creating safe transitions for patients with VTE. Process metrics such as patient and/or family education occurred successfully in 1,013 cases, follow-up phone calls occurred in 810 cases, and medication reconciliation occurred in 1,182 patients across all cohorts. Outcome metrics such as readmission rate were 3.8% across the cohorts and were attributed to the development of major bleeding or recurrent VTE. Emergency Department utilization was 4.8%. Finally, access to medications was not a cause for readmissions or recurrent VTE.[25] It should be noted that this program was started and implemented during the COVID-19 pandemic, which greatly impacted available resources and support. Programs such as SHM FAST offer a focused transition plan for patients with VTE.

SUMMARY

In conclusion, patients transitioning from the hospital setting with VTE are vulnerable due to multiple factors inherent in current care models. The concern over adverse drug events associated with anticoagulation potentially leading to re-hospitalization and harm deserves special attention. Nonetheless, many models provide only limited attention to the VTE patient. There are new and innovative programs, such as SHM FAST, that specifically target this patient population. Further investigation and widespread implementation strategies are needed to improve this process and create a safe transition for patients with VTE.

CLINICS CARE POINTS

- Patients transitioning from the hospital setting are vulnerable to harm.
- There are new and innovative strategies designed to create safe transitions.

DISCLOSURE

AJM was a mentor for the Society of Hospital Medicine.

REFERENCES

1. CDC Data and Statistics on Venous Thromboembolism. Available at: https://www. cdc.gov/ncbddd/dvt/ha-vte.html. Last Accessed February 26, 2023.
2. Grosse SD, Nelson RE, Nyarko KA, et al. The economic burden of incident venous thromboembolism in the United States: a review of estimated attributable healthcare costs. Thromb Res 2016;137:3–10.
3. Kripalani S, LeFevre F, Phillips CO, et al. Deficits and communication and information transfer between hospital-based and primary care physicians: implications for patient safety and continuity of care. JAMA 2007;297(8):831–41.
4. Schillinger D, Piette J, Grumbach K, et al. Closing the loop: physician communication with diabetic patients who have low health literacy. Arch Intern Med 2003; 163:83–90.
5. Coffey C, Greenwald J, Budnitz T, et al. Project BOOST® Implementation Guide. second edition. The Society of Hospital Medicine; 2013.
6. Roy CL, Poon EG, Karson AS, et al. Patient safety concerns arising from test results that return after hospital discharge. Ann Intern Med 2005;143(2):121–8.
7. Were MC, Li X, Kesterson J, et al. Adequacy of hospital discharge summaries in documenting tests with pending results and outpatient follow-up providers. J Gen Intern Med 2009;24(9):1002–6.
8. Walz SE, Smith M, Cox E, et al. Pending laboratory tests and the hospital discharge summary in patients discharged to sub-acute care. J Gen Intern Med 2011;26(4):393–8.
9. Budnitz DS, Lovegove MC, Shehab N, et al. Emergency hospitalizations for adverse drug events in older americans. NEJM 2011;365:2002–12.
10. Stevens SM, Woller SC, Baumann Kreuzinger L, et al. Antithrombotic therapy for VTE disease second update of the chest guideline and expert panel report. Chest 2021;160(6):e545–608.
11. Ortel TL, Neuman I, Ageno W, et al. American Society of Hematology 2020 guidelines for management of venous thromboembolism: treatment of deep vein thrombosis and pulmonary embolism. Blood Advances 2020;4(19):4693–738.
12. Aujesky D, Obrosky DS, Stone RA, et al. Derivation and validation of a prognostic model for pulmonary embolism. Am J Respir Crit Care Med 2005;172(8):1041–6.
13. Jimenez D, Aujesky D, Moores L, et al. RIETE Investigators. Simplification of the pulmonary embolism severity index for prognostication in patients with acute symptomatic pulmonary embolism. Arch Intern Med 2010;170(15):1383–9.
14. Zondag W, Mos ICM, Creemers-Schild D, et al. Outpatient treatment in patients with acute pulmonary embolism: the Hestia study. J Thromb Haemost 2011; 9(8):1500–7.
15. Bova C, Sanchez O, Prandoni P, et al. Identification of intermediate-risk patients with acute symptomatic pulmonary embolism. Eur Respir J 2014;44(3):694–703.
16. R3 report issue 19: National patient safety goal for anticoagulant therapy. Available at: https://www.jointcommission.org/r3_report_issue_19_national_patient_safety_goal_for_anticoagulant_therapy. Accessed February 26, 2023.
17. Donzé J, Aujesky D, Williams D, et al. Potentially avoidable 30-day hospital readmissions in medical patients: derivation and validation of a prediction model. JAMA Intern Med 2013;173(8):632–8.
18. Van Walraven C, Dhalia IA, Bell C, et al. Derivation and validation of an index to predict early death or unplanned readmission after discharge from hospital to the community. CMAJ (Can Med Assoc J) 2010;182(6):551–7.

19. Charlson ME, Pompei P, Ales KL, et al. A new method of classifying prognostic comorbidity in longitudinal studies: development and validation. J Chronic Dis 1987;40:373.
20. Karaoui LR, Ramia E, Mansour H, et al. Impact of pharmacist-conducted anticoagulation patient education and telephone follow-up on transitions of care: a randomized controlled trial. BMC Health Serv Res 2021;21:151.
21. Zdyb EG impact of discharge anticoagulation education by emergency department pharmacists at a tertiary academic medical center. The Journal of Emergency Medicine 2017;53(6):896–903.
22. Sanchez GM, Douglass MA, Mancuso M. Revisiting project re-engineered discharge (RED): the impact of a pharmacist telephone intervention on hospital readmission rates. Pharmacotherapy 2015;35(9):805–12.
23. Merli G, Hiestand B, Amin A, et al. Balancing anti-thrombotic efficacy and bleeding risk in the contemporary management of venous thromboembolism. Curr Emerg Hosp Med Rep 2015;389–99.
24. Galanis T, Thomson L, Orapallo D, et al. Society of Hospital Medicine Facilitation of Anticoagulation for Safer Transitions Program Implementation Guide. 2022.
25. Internal data presented at SHM FAST presentation September 22,2022.

Varicose Veins

Approach, Assessment, and Management to the Patient with Chronic Venous Disease

Viviane Seki Sassaki, MD, RPVI, RVT, RDMS[a], Eri Fukaya, MD, PhD[b],*

KEYWORDS

- Varicose veins • Chronic venous disease • Pelvic congestion disorders
- Postthrombotic syndrome

KEY POINTS

- Varicose veins is a common presentation of chronic venous disease but there are many other signs and symptoms associated.
- Venous hypertension is the underlying pathologic condition of chronic venous disease.
- It is important to understand the pathophysiology, risk factors, differential diagnosis workup, and prognosis to provide appropriate treatment.
- Clinical assessment for the assessment of chronic venous disease is very important because diagnostic testing results and symptoms do not always correlate.

INTRODUCTION

Varicose veins is a common condition affecting more than 25 million people in the United States.[1] The development of varicose veins involves a complex and multifactorial interplay between the genetic makeup of the individual and predisposing risk factors such as age, female sex, family history, pregnancy, obesity, and prolonged standing. Persistent venous hypertension and the consequences of chronic inflammation within the venous wall are contributory factors for varicose vein development. Important to note is that varicose veins is one manifestation of a spectrum of disease called chronic venous disease. The aim of this article is to review the approach to the patient with chronic venous disease and highlight its management strategies.

LOWER EXTREMITY VENOUS ANATOMY AND PATHOPHYSIOLOGY

The veins of the lower extremity are a networked formation of both superficial and deep veins, with mutual connections, such as tributaries or accessories and perforators.

[a] Stanford Heart and Vascular Clinic- Vascular Laboratory, Stanford, CA 94305, USA; [b] Division of Vascular Surgery, Stanford University School of Medicine, Stanford, CA, USA
* Corresponding author. 780 Welch Road, Suite CJ 350, Palo Alto, CA 94304.
E-mail address: efukaya@stanford.edu

Med Clin N Am 107 (2023) 895–909
https://doi.org/10.1016/j.mcna.2023.05.002
0025-7125/23/© 2023 Elsevier Inc. All rights reserved.

The deep venous system is bordered by the *fascia muscularis* and is composed of the femoral, common femoral, and deep femoral veins and the popliteal, peroneal, tibial, soleus, and gastrocnemius veins (GAV). The main function of the deep system is to transport venous blood toward the heart. Most of the lower extremity venous blood resides in the deep veins. The superficial venous system is situated superficial to the deep fascia, either in the fascial plane or in the subcutaneous tissue. It consists of the great and small saphenous veins (SSVs), anterior accessory saphenous, posterior accessory saphenous, and its tributaries (**Fig. 1**). Classified more generally as the axial superficial veins, the great saphenous vein (GSV) and SSV connect to the deep system through the saphenofemoral junction (SFJ) and saphenopopliteal junction (SPJ), respectively. The SFJ has 2 valves. The terminal valve is located at the common femoral vein confluence and the preterminal valve is caudad to the terminal valve and adjacent to its other branches, such as the epigastric, pudendal, and circumflex veins. The other axial vein confluence is the SPJ, where the SSV connects to the deep venous system through the popliteal vein (POPV). However, there can be anatomical variation where it extends cranially above the knee before connecting to the deep venous system. Anatomical variants where the cranial extension connects to the GSV are known as the intersaphenous vein (commonly called the vein of Giacomini). Tributary veins, which are the branch veins can drain into the deep or superficial venous system, are often associated with varicose veins. The anterior accessory saphenous vein (AASV) runs anteriorly in the lower extremity and the posterior accessory saphenous vein courses on the medial posterior side. The difference between prominent tributaries from the saphenous vein can be elucidated with anatomical landmarks.

The bridge between the superficial system and the deep venous system is through perforator veins, which conduct from the superficial to the deep system.

Most anatomical variations are duplicative and/or segmental; however, a completely duplicative system seems rare.

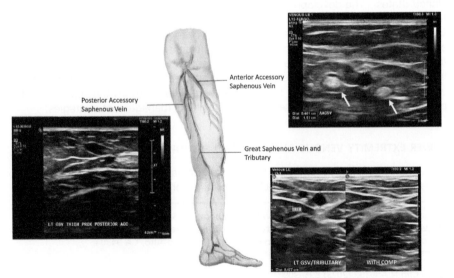

Fig. 1. Superficial venous system visualized during ultrasound testing. AASV within lymph nodes (*arrows*) as landmarks for identification.

The lower extremity venous system is responsible for the unidirectional venous return to the inferior vena cava and can be observed using ultrasound. This venous return occurs during the diastolic cycle, aided by intravenous valve compression often with the aid of calf muscle contraction. However, if this flow balance is disrupted and changes the venous blood flow direction, some of the blood that should have forward flow will remain in the veins creating venous hypertension. This can cause inflammation in the vessel walls resulting in vessel wall changes and superficial venous system dilatation (mostly tributaries), aka varicose veins, and other structural changes that also lead to clinical symptoms.

CLASSIFICATION OF VENOUS DISEASE

Venous disease can be due to venous hypertension or thrombosis. What we refer to as chronic venous disease is due to hypertension although there can be an overlap with venous thrombosis because this can cause venous hypertension. Chronic venous disease is often of primary cause but can also have other underlying causes such as post-thrombotic syndrome (PTS) and pelvic venous disorders (PeVDs). In addition, there are disorders such as lymphedema and lipedema, which can often be misdiagnosed as chronic venous disease due to disease overlap and similar presentation and appearances.

Chronic Venous Disease

Chronic venous disease can interfere with quality of life due to pain, reduced mobility, and reduced work ability. Symptoms usually result from venous hypertension caused by circulatory reflux and/or venous obstruction and can have a wide range of presentations, including varicose veins, edema, skin changes, and/or venous leg ulcers.[2] Varicose veins are one the most common manifestations of chronic venous disease and is characterized by tortuous and dilated veins. Symptoms can vary significantly, with some of these being asymptomatic to those associated with pain, itching, heaviness, burning, and swelling. With more advanced venous disease, in addition to varicose veins, there can be dermatological changes including skin pigmentation and ulcerations.[3]

Venous dysfunction can be congenital, primary, or secondary. For example, some congenital disorders are associated with varicose veins, whereas primary varicose veins are the result of a progressive increase in the elasticity and valvular incompetency of the veins with progressive vessel dilatation.[4] Secondary varicose veins occur due to venous hypertension as a consequence of deep venous outflow obstruction causing back pressure (such as PTS).[5]

Chronic venous disease is described using the Clinical-Etiologic-Anatomic-Physiologic (CEAP) classification (**Table 1**), originally published in 1995 and revised in 2020.[6] Using this classification, patients can be arranged based on clinical, etiological, and pathophysiological manifestations. Chronic venous insufficiency refers to the more advanced form of the chronic venous disease, which is CEAP C4 to C6, which may or may not be associated with varicose veins. In addition to the CEAP classification, the Venous Clinical Severity Score (VCSS) is a tool to evaluate clinical symptoms and can change with the progression of disease and treatment (**Table 2**). The VCSS ranges from 0 to 30 points by evaluating 10 clinical items as none (0), mild (1), moderate (2), and severe (3).

Deep Vein Thrombosis and Post Thrombotic Syndrome

Venous thromboembolism disorders, including deep vein thrombosis (DVT) and pulmonary embolism. Residual thrombus and scarring of the deep veins due to earlier DVT can cause PTS. PTS causes venous hypertension distally and commonly presents in the lower extremities as debilitating symptoms including continued pain,

Table 1
Clinical-etiologic-anatomic-physiologic classification

Clinical	Etiological	Anatomical	Pathophysiologic
C0: no venous or palpable signs of venous disease	Ep: Primary	As: Telangiectasia (Tel), reticular veins (Ret), GSV above knee (GSVa), GSV below Knee (GSVb), SSV, AASV, Nonsaphenous vein	Pr: Reflux
C1: Telangiectasias and/or reticular veins (<3 mm in diameter)	Es: Secondary	Ap: Thigh perforator, calf perforator	Po: Obstruction
C2: Varicose veins (≥3 mm in diameter)	Esi: Secondary Intravenous	Ad: IVC, CIV, IIV, EIV, PELV, CFV, DFV, FV, POPV, tibial vein, peroneal vein, ATV, PTV, muscular veins, GAV, Soleal vein (SOV)	Pro: Reflux and obstruction
C2r: Recurrent varicose veins	Ese: Secondary extravenous	An: No venous anatomy identified	Pn: No venous pathophysiology identified
C3: Edema	Ec: Congenital		
C4: Skin and subcutaneous tissue changes, secondary to CVD	En: No cause identified		
C4a: Pigmentation or eczema			
C4b: Lipodermatosclerosis or atrophie blanche			
C4c: Corona Phlebectatica			
C5: Healed			
C6: Active venous ulcers			
C6r: Recurrent active venous ulcers			

Abbreviations: ATV, anterior tibial vein; CFV, common femoral vein; DFV, deep femoral vein; FV, femoral vein; PTV, posterior tibial vein.

Table 2
Venous clinical severity score

Pain or other discomfort (aching, heaviness, fatigue, soreness, burning)	Induration Includes white atrophy and lipodermatosclerosis
None: 0	None: 0
Mild: 1 Occasional pain or other discomfort	Mild: 1 Limited to perimalleolar area
Moderate: 2 Daily pain or other discomfort	Moderate: 2 Diffuse over lower third of calf
Severe: 3 Daily pain or discomfort	Severe: 3 Wider distributions above lower third of calf
Varicose veins	*Active ulcer number*
None: 0	None: 0
Mild: 1 Few and scattered	Mild: 1
Moderate: 2 Confined to calf or thigh	Moderate: 2
Severe: 3 Involves calf and thigh	Severe: ≥3
Venous edema	
None: 0	Active ulcer duration (longest active)
Mild: 1 Limited to foot and ankle area	1. <3 mo
Moderate: 2 Extends above ankle but below knee	2. >3 mo but <1 y
Severe: 3 Extends to knee and above	3. Not healed for >1 y
Skin pigmentation	Active ulcer size (largest active)
None: 0 None or focal	4. Diameter <2 cm
Mild: 1 Limited to perimalleolar area	5. Diameter 2–6 cm
Moderate: 2 Diffuse over lower third of calf	6. Diameter >6 cm
Severe: 3 Wider distribution above lower third of calf	
Inflammation (erythema, cellulitis, venous eczema, dermatitis)	*Use of compression therapy*
None: 0	0 Not used
Mild: 1 Limited to perimalleolar area	1 Intermittent use of stockings
Moderate: 2 Diffuse over lower third of calf	2 Wears stockings most days
Severe: 3 Wider distribution above lower third of calf	3 Full compliance

edema, skin changes, and venous leg ulcers due to venous stasis.[7–9] PTS is a highly morbid complication of DVT and has been quoted to be as high as 40% to 50% of the cases due to either residual venous obstruction or venous valve damage.[9] The most severe PTS cases including those with venous ulcers occur in 5% to 10% of patients.[9] The clinical presentation of a PTS may resemble primary venous insufficiency such as leg pain, fatigue, limb swelling, and lower limb heaviness sensation, and one needs to consider this by obtaining a history of DVT and also carefully examining the ultrasound images. The symptomatology usually accentuates during prolonged standing-up, noticeably at the end of the day or during ambulation. There is no classification of PTS despite the wide spectrum of disease. However, the Villalta score (**Table 3**), which is composed of clinical and physiologic indices specifically for PTS can be used to evaluate severity. The score gives points for symptoms, clinical signs, and severity of the disease. In the presence of any ulcer, it is classified as severe, even if no other signs or symptoms are present.[10]

Table 3
Villalta score for postthrombotic syndrome classification

Symptoms/Clinical Signs	None	Mild	Moderate	Severe
Symptoms				
Pain	0	1	2	3
Cramps	0	1	2	3
Heaviness	0	1	2	3
Paresthesia	0	1	2	3
Pruritus	0	1	2	3
Clinical Signs				
Pretibial edema	0	1	2	3
Skin induration	0	1	2	3
Hyperpigmentation	0	1	2	3
Redness	0	1	2	3
Venous ectasia	0	1	2	3
Pain on calf compression	0	1	2	3
Venous Ulcer	Absent			Present

Pelvic Venous Disorders

Most lower extremity chronic venous disease stems from disease distal to the external iliac veins. However, there can be venous disease from the internal iliac veins or other abdominal and pelvic veins (PELV). This is defined as PeVDs and can present with a constellation of symptoms (abdominal bloating, dyspareunia, bladder and bowel symptoms, and so forth) often described as pelvic congestion syndrome. Atypical varicosities, such as those seen at the vulvar or that course along the posterior thigh from the groin, may indicate PeVD. The pelvic varicosities are associated with primary reflux in the ovarian, internal iliac vein and obstruction of left renal or common iliac veins, and are often the cause of increased pressures causing venous dilations and chronic pelvic pain. Compression of the left renal vein, known as Nutcracker syndrome, can cause left flank pain, abdominal pain, and hematuria.

The relationship between pelvic symptoms and venous pathologic condition is far more complex than in the lower extremities. Various symptoms can associate with different pathophysiologic mechanisms of compression and obstruction. In addition, the symptoms can be due to interchangeable origin. It is important to classify PeVDs for proper patient management and future clinical research. Categorization based on the symptoms-varices-pathophysiology (SVP) of pelvic venous disorders has a similar structure to the CEAP classification. The use of the SVP classification provides a common language to discuss the disease correctly reducing possibilities for conceivable misdiagnosis, suboptimal treatment, and undesirable patient outcomes.[11]

Lipedema and Phlebolymphedema

Commonly encountered differential diagnoses for chronic venous disease are phlebolymphedema and lipedema because patients present with complaints of "swelling" in both conditions. Patients with lipedema are seen frequently in the vascular clinical practice because they can be confused with lymphedema or chronic venous disease. Lipedema is characterized by abnormal fat tissue deposition. This can occur both in the upper and lower extremities and including the trunk but mostly seen in the bilateral calves, thighs, and gluteal region. It is associated with orthostatic edema and pain. The trigger mechanism for fat distribution disorder is still unknown.[12] In conjunction with clinical assessment characterized by the symmetric lobulated fat disproportion seen in the bilateral lower extremities,[13] female sex exclusivity, family history, the onset of fat accumulation (usually during puberty), lack of success with diet and exercise, and clothing size difference between the affected areas versus not (can often have more than a 2-size difference) can help with the lipedema diagnosis. Physical symptoms can range from bilateral lower extremity pain, sensitivity to touch, sensations of heaviness or burning, and easy bruising (**Fig. 2**). The diagnosis is one of clinical judgment, and there are no tests to diagnose lipedema.[14] Therefore, misdiagnosis can often occur, causing patient grief.[15] The consensus document from the International Union of Phlebology suggests a classification depending on the location of the fat deposits.[16,17]

Phlebolymphedema occurs when the lymphatic system is compromised due to a congenital or acquired lymphatic fluid transportation insufficiency. The extremities are most often affected but other parts of the human body can be affected, such as the head, neck, torso, and genital region. Patient's history and physical examination will usually be sufficient to make the diagnosis. However, further imaging can be warranted in cases where proximal obstruction of the vein or lymphatics is suspected. Examinations such as lymphangiography and functional lymph scintigraphy can also contribute to identifying lymphatic dysfunction. Different from lipedema, lymphedema is more often unilateral. In addition, it affects both men and women along with dermatologic system compromise.[18] When there is an overlap of chronic venous disease and lymphedema, this is called phlebolymphedema. Even though newer surgical techniques to reconstruct the lymphatic vein anastomosis to lymph nodes and vessel transplantation can be considered, conservative treatment remains predominant with compression, lymphatic drainage, and skin care.

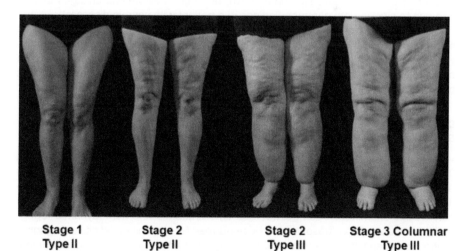

| Stage 1 | Stage 2 | Stage 2 | Stage 3 Columnar |
| Type II | Type II | Type III | Type III |

Fig. 2. Stages of Lipedema from Herbst KL. Subcutaneous Adipose Tissue Diseases: Dercum Disease, Lipedema, Familial Multiple Lipomatosis, and Madelung Disease. [Updated 2019 Dec 14]. In: Feingold KR, Anawalt B, Blackman MR, et al., editors. Endotext [Internet]. South Dartmouth (MA): MDText.com, Inc.; 2000.

Central Venous Hypertension

Extravascular causes for venous hypertension include increased central pressures (obesity, right heart failure, pulmonary hypertension, atrial fibrillation, significant tricuspid valve regurgitation, and pelvic congestion), anatomical compression (May Thurner syndrome and Nutcracker syndrome), and tumor compression. The mere existence of venous hypertension does not necessarily cause venous symptoms but can trigger this by inciting factors such as pressure, causing venous obstruction, inflammation (cellulitis), or trauma.

APPROACH TO THE PATIENT WITH VENOUS DISEASE

The anamnesis for patients with venous disease reflects venous hypertension due to venous reflux and/or venous obstruction. The presentation ranges from asymptomatic spider veins to severely debilitating conditions such as nonhealing ulcers. Evaluating the patient's signs and symptoms is essential to correctly identify that it is due to vein pathologic condition. Information regarding the history of earlier surgeries, medical conditions, trauma, and occupation (due to an orthostatic component) should always be investigated. History taking should include assessment for risk factors, including age, sex, body habitus, sedentarism, pregnancy history, familiar history, occupation, and exercise habits. In addition to earlier history and treatment of venous disease, DVT, thrombophlebitis, medications, and other underlying medical problems are also pertinent to the approach in a patient with venous disease.

Symptoms may aggravate toward the end of the day, during prolonged orthostatism, during heat, and amid the premenstrual phase for women. Symptoms usually improve when the patient elevates their lower limbs and with limb movement. During the physical examination, in addition to the leg examination, it is important to note if there are any varicosities in the abdomen or the vulva area (for women). Skin changes including discoloration (hemosiderin staining), scarred tissue (atrophie blanche), dilated reticular veins at the ankles and foot (corona phlebectatica), texture change (lipodermatosclerosis) and skin breakdown, or wounds as well as changes in limb size due to swelling are common findings in a patient with venous disease.

A patient with chronic venous disease should be evaluated in an upright position as much as possible. This is because there is a significant effect of gravity and weight on venous return. To minimize these effects, the examination should be performed in a bright environment and after some minutes while a patient stands up, bearing weight on the contralateral lower extremity.[19]

DIAGNOSTIC EVALUATION
Duplex Ultrasound Examination

Venous duplex ultrasound evaluation should be performed to identify and characterize the cause of venous insufficiency (venous insufficiency is synonymous with venous reflux). Although this is not a direct measurement of the underlying pathologic condition of venous hypertension, it may help to elicit the mechanism causing this. This noninvasive examination can provide real-time anatomic and hemodynamic topography. Venous duplex ultrasound can be performed for screening, definitive diagnosis, pretreatment and peri-interventional mapping, procedural guidance, posttreatment site inspection, and long-term follow-up. A comprehensive venous duplex ultrasound examination consists of the evaluation for acute or chronic thrombosis (including PTS) causing obstruction and the insufficiency of venous valves in both the deep and superficial veins. Ultrasound scanning can usually be readily done for below the inguinal ligament but for the ilio-caval system, the ability to perform sufficient examination will depend significantly on the patient's body habitus. Ultrasound may not offer proper diagnosis given it will lose resolution when attempting to image at such depth.

Ultrasound findings can assist on determining venous size, anatomical variation, incompressibility, echogenicity, and vessel patency (**Fig. 3**). Normal venous flow on ultrasound should be spontaneous and respirophasic (responds to respiration) and, unidirectional toward heart with good response to proximal or distal augmentation (normal response is absence of flow). During examination, the patient should be positioned in a steep reversed Trendelenburg or in the standing up position to best simulate physiologic conditions. The axial venous flow will be evaluated in the superficial and deep venous system, testing the capability of proper valve closure at the SFJ, thigh, knee, and calf. The documentation of GSV, SSV, and main tributaries consists of vessel caliber, depth from the skin, and reflux time.

In patients presenting with open wounds and a history of an earlier venous ablation and or stripping, it is important to demonstrate incompetent perforators associated with varicose veins toward the wound area. For these patients, the evaluation consists of documenting possible sources of venous compromise by targeting areas adjacent to the wound. The subcutaneous tissue on ultrasound will demonstrate the presence of edema or adipose tissue accumulation and can help to identify lipedema and lymphedema, which will differ by its echogenicity. Edema usually seems as trabeculated hypoechoic and echogenic areas, whereas fat seems diffusely echogenic due to sound attenuation (**Fig. 4**).

An evaluation for obstruction will proceed testing for valvular insufficiency. Following evaluation for compressibility, the assessment for retrograde flow (reflux) is performed with the use of Valsalva and other augmentation maneuvers. The venous valve closure time is known as reflux, and this represents the flow going the opposite direction of physiologic normal venous flow. The refluxing time is obtained while acquiring the Doppler spectral waveforms and interpreting color flow orientation. If the deep venous presents valvular closure more than 1.0 seconds, the patient has a positive test for deep venous insufficiency (**Fig. 5**). Venous reflux times do not correlate with chronic venous disease severity.[20] This is because venous reflux time does not always correlate with venous hypertension. A reflux of more than 0.5 seconds is considered a positive test in the superficial venous system. This is tested for in all segments of the GSV and SSV, including the SPJ and SFJ in the lower extremity. Venous insufficiency can be segmental or involve the entire vein. Any observed retrograde flow may be explained by tributary confluence entering the main saphenous vein, a valve leakage due to improper anatomical or physiologic closure dysfunction, and residual from surgical correction to preserve drainage.

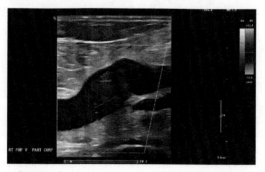

Fig. 3. Enlargement of POPV during acute nonocclusive deep venous thrombosis.

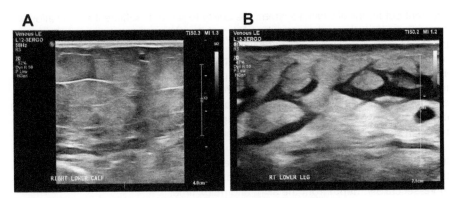

Fig. 4. Ultrasound imaging of lymphedema (A) and lipedema (B).

Computed Tomography and Magnetic Resonance (MR) Venogram

Evaluating the abdominal and pelvic venous structures with ultrasound can be challenging due to bowel gas shadowing, technical difficulty, vessel anatomy, and body habitus. Computed tomography venography (CTV) and magnetic resonance venography (MRV) are the imaging of choice for venous imaging in the abdomen and pelvis. This imaging will describe the general venous anatomy and provide information on enlarged lymph nodes or tumors that can cause a mass effect and/or obstruction. In addition, the imaging of adjacent structures can aid in diagnosing soft tissue and bone abnormalities seen in association with vascular malformation syndromes such as *Klippel-Trénaunay* syndrome, unusual anatomic causes of varicose veins, congenital venous malformation, and portosystemic collateral-related varicose vein pathologic conditions.[21] Although CTV and MRV can provide excellent images with good spatial resolution, the requirement of patients to be in a prone position for the examination can often disguise the physiological effects that gravity and weight can have on venous disease. In addition, it cannot provide hemodynamic information, so can be difficult to detect the presence of reflux.

Venogram and Intravascular Ultrasound

The need for diagnostic venography in patients with varicose veins has decreased significantly due to ultrasound advancements as being less invasive and relaying on

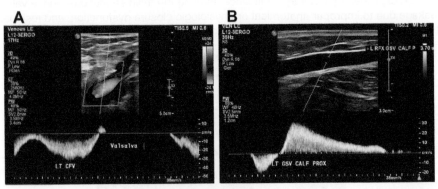

Fig. 5. (A) No evidence of deep venous insufficiency during Valsalva maneuver, (B) Superficial venous insufficiency seen in the GSV with reflux of 3.7s after proper distal augmentation.

visualization of vessel walls and direction of flow. Venography is more commonly performed in the setting of endovenous intervention[22] and consists of contrast injection by a syringe or mechanical-pressure injectors with dynamic fluoroscopy examination. Intravascular ultrasound (IVUS) aims to acquire real-time cross-sectional anatomy. The vessel lumen and walls are visualized, leading to superior diagnostic information. IVUS can be more sensitive for assessing iliofemoral vein stenosis than venography and frequently leads to revised treatment plans and the potential for improved clinical outcomes.[23] However, IVUS examination is more sensitive than venography.[24] Venography with IVUS can be helpful for occasional cases with inconclusive ultrasound, CTV, or MRV imaging. The procedure can also treat endovascularly venous obstruction.[25] A study comparing descending venography and duplex ultrasound demonstrated that duplex examination reflects the degree and distribution of venous reflux more accurately compared with descending venography.[26]

Plethysmography

Plethysmography is the evaluation of flow through luminous infrared reflection from capillaries. Although plethysmography is not routinely used in venous care, it provides volume variation accordingly to the amount of blood flow return. A normal venous refilling time can be considered less than 20 seconds without a tourniquet. The refilling time of more than 20 seconds with a tourniquet is compatible with GSV incompetence.[27] A study reported that the use of plethysmography with provocative maneuvers might be appropriate for assessing venous insufficiency. However, it was not recommended for acute deep venous thrombosis.[28,29]

MANAGEMENT

The goal in the treatment of chronic venous disease is to resolve symptoms that reduce quality of life (QOL), heal venous leg ulcers if these are present, prevent bleeding, or reduce the recurrence of thrombophlebitis. The treatment of symptomatic and advanced chronic venous disease are considered medical treatment, whereas treatment of asymptomatic C1 and C2 disease is considered chiefly cosmetic. Treatment modalities include conservative therapies such as compression therapy, venotonic medications, and venous procedures, including sclerotherapy, surgical therapy, and endovenous therapies.

Compression Therapy

Compression therapy aims to counteract venous hypertension caused by incompetent valves and other causes, thereby reducing edema. Compression is used to treat swelling, symptomatic varicose veins, and venous ulcers. The most common form of compression is elastic socks/stockings, elastic and nonelastic multilayer wraps, and intermittent pneumatic compression (IPC). IPC is a mechanical method of delivering compression to swollen limbs by applying a multichamber compression sleeve over the affected limb and sequentially inflating and deflating the device to apply sustained pressure, proving a venous milking effect. For patients with venous ulcers or excessive swelling, the Unna boot, which is a zinc oxide short stretch multilayer wrap provides excellent compression and has been shown to accelerate the venous ulcer healing process.

Medical Therapy

Venoactive drugs can be used for symptom alleviation. Micronized purified flavonoid fraction has been studied and found to prevent endothelial activation and inflammation, thereby slowing venous reflux and its clinical sequelae, such as leg heaviness, swelling, and cramps.[30] Some randomized clinical trials (RCTs) have also shown other flavonoids, including red grapeseed extract, horse chestnut seed extract, and diosmin, to be effective at reducing edema, pain, and itching.

Sclerotherapy

Sclerotherapy is an effective method to destroy and close incompetent veins. It involves injection of a chemical agent into the lumen of a vessel in order to induce damage and occlusion of the vessel. Vein sclerosing is achieved through direct injection of liquid or foamed agents to provoke endothelial cell and vessel wall damage.

Sclerotherapy is used for the treatment of varicose veins, incompetent veins, reticular veins, and spider veins.[31]

Endovenous Treatment

Catheter-based ablations include thermal and nonthermal ablation options. Endovenous thermal ablation uses ultrasound-guided, catheter-directed thermal energy to cause endothelial damage causing the vein wall to contract and occlude. The 2 thermal options are endovenous laser ablation and radiofrequency ablation. Endovenous thermal ablations are the treatment of choice for saphenous incompetence, and most current evidence supports that ablation of an incompetent superficial venous system promotes ulcer healing and prevents ulcer recurrence.[32,33]

The nonthermal, endovenous treatment includes the use of cyanoacrylate glue and mechanochemical ablation. The VenaSeal (Medtronic, MN) technology dispenses cyanoacrylate glue from the catheter tip to occlude or "seal" the refluxing truncal superficial veins to treat varicose veins and venous insufficiency.[34] Mechanochemical endovenous ablation uses a rotating wire within a catheter to mechanically damage the endothelium of a vessel while, at the same time, a sclerosant is infused at the end of the catheter, which causes chemical damage to the same segment of vein wall.[35]

Surgical Treatment

For surgical treatment, high ligation with or without stripping of the saphenous vein have been used historically. However, more recently, endovenous therapy have become the main therapy option, and these surgical techniques are mostly used in cases when there is a contraindication to endovenous treatment.

Ambulatory phlebectomy is a safe and effective procedure that includes the removal of varicose veins through small incisions in the leg and can be done under local anesthesia in an office setting.

PROGNOSIS

Chronic venous disease, as the name implies, is a chronic disease and is usually not curative. Despite adequate preventative measures or treatment, there is a high incidence of disease progression or recurrence because there is a component of natural aging and cumulative venous pressures on the venous system. Thus, the goal of treatment of chronic venous disease should be to perform treatment of the bothersome symptom or presentation for the patient and not to focus on treating imaging findings.

CLINICS CARE POINTS

- Deep vein thrombosis and associated post thrombotic syndrome, pelvic venous disorder and lymphedema can overlap with and present as chronic venous disease.
- Recognizing these conditions are an important part of the clinical work up.

DISCLOSURE

The authors have nothing to disclose.

REFERENCES

1. Beebe-Dimmer JL, Pfeifer JR, Engle JS, et al. The epidemiology of chronic venous insufficiency and varicose veins. Ann Epidemiol 2005;15(3):175–84.
2. Eberhardt RT, Raffetto JD. Chronic venous insufficiency. Circulation 2014;130(4): 333–46.
3. Gawas M, Bains A, Janghu S, et al. A Comprehensive Review on Varicose Veins: Preventive Measures and Different Treatments. J Am Nutr Assoc 2022;41(5): 499–510.
4. Boivin P, Cornu-Thenard A, Charpak Y. Pregnancy-induced changes in lower extremity superficial veins: an ultrasound scan study. J Vasc Surg 2000;32(3): 570–4.
5. Álvarez LNG, Sánchez CA, Pérez QCL. Prevalencia de insuficiencia venosa en jóvenes universitarios y factores de riesgo correlacionados con el estadio clínico (ceap c 1 y 2). Dermatología Cosmética, Médica y Quirúrgica 2017;15(4):222–6.
6. Lurie F, Passman M, Meisner M, et al. The 2020 update of the CEAP classification system and reporting standards. J Vasc Surg Venous Lymphat Disord 2020;8(3): 342–52 [Erratum in: J Vasc Surg Venous Lymphat Disord. 2021;9(1):288].
7. Khan SR. The Post-thrombotic syndrome. Hematology Am Soc Hematol Educ Program 2016;2016(1):413–8.
8. Fletcher-Sanfeliu D, Redón J, García-Granero Á, et al. 'Pulmonary thrombosis in situ': risk factors, clinic characteristics and long-term evolution. Blood Coagul Fibrinolysis 2020;31(7):469–75.
9. Cosmi B, Stanek A, Kozak M, et al. The Post-thrombotic Syndrome-Prevention and Treatment: VAS-European Independent Foundation in Angiology/Vascular Medicine Position Paper. Front Cardiovasc Med 2022;9:762443.
10. Villalta S, Bagatella P, Piccioli A, et al. Assessment of validity and reproducibility of a clinical scale for the post thrombotic syndrome. Haemostasis 1994;24:158a.
11. Meissner MH, Khilnani NM, Labropoulos N, et al. The Symptoms-Varices-Pathophysiology classification of pelvic venous disorders: A report of the American Vein & Lymphatic Society International Working Group on Pelvic Venous Disorders. J Vasc Surg Venous Lymphat Disord 2021;9(3):568–84.
12. Jandali Z, Merwart B, Jiga L. The Lipedema. In: Jandali Z, Jiga LP, Campisi C, editors. Lipedema. Cham: Springer; 2022. https://doi.org/10.1007/978-3-030-86 717-1_1.
13. Fife CE, Maus EA, Carter MJ. Lipedema: a frequently misdiagnosed and misunderstood fatty deposition syndrome. Adv Skin Wound Care 2010;23(2):81–92 [quiz: 93–4].
14. Kruppa P, Georgiou I, Biermann N, et al. Lipedema-Pathogenesis, Diagnosis, and Treatment Options. Dtsch Arztebl Int 2020;117(22–23):396–403.

15. Clarke C, Kirby JN, Smidt T, et al. Stages of lipoedema: experiences of physical and mental health and health care. Qual Life Res 2022. https://doi.org/10.1007/s11136-022-03216-w.

16. Wollina U, Heinig B. Differenzialdiagnostik von Lipödem und Lymphödem : Ein Leitfaden für die Praxis [Differential diagnostics of lipedema and lymphedema: A practical guideline]. Hautarzt 2018;69(12):1039–47. German.

17. Lee BB, Andrade M, Antignani PL, et al. International Union of Phlebology. Diagnosis and treatment of primary lymphedema. Consensus document of the International Union of Phlebology (IUP)-2013. Int Angiol 2013;32(6):541–74.

18. Amato ACM, Amato FCM, Amato JLS, et al. Lipedema prevalence and risk factors in Brazil. J Vasc Bras 2022. https://doi.org/10.1590/1677-5449.202101981. 21e20210198.

19. Baliyan V, Tajmir S, Hedgire SS, et al. Lower extremity venous reflux. Cardiovasc Diagn Ther 2016;6(6):533–43.

20. Yamaki T, Nozaki M, Sasaki K. Quantitative assessment of superficial venous insufficiency using duplex ultrasound and air plethysmography. Dermatol Surg 2000;26(7):644–8.

21. Bandali MF, Mirakhur A, Lee EW, et al. Portal hypertension: Imaging of portosystemic collateral pathways and associated image-guided therapy. World J Gastroenterol 2017;23(10):1735–46.

22. Varicose Veins Aditya Sharma and Suman Wasan in Vascular Medicine: A Companion to Braunwald's Heart Disease, 53, 693-708 edition 2020.

23. Saleem T, Knight A, Raju S. Diagnostic yield of intravascular ultrasound in patients with clinical signs and symptoms of lower extremity venous disease. J Vasc Surg Venous Lymphat Disord 2020;8(4):634–9.

24. Montminy ML, Thomasson JD, Tanaka GJ, et al. A comparison between intravascular ultrasound and venography in identifying key parameters essential for iliac vein stenting. J Vasc Surg Venous Lymphat Disord 2019;7(6):801–7.

25. Creager MA, Beckman JA and Loscalzo J. Vascular medicine: a companion to braunwald's heart disease, 2020, Elsevier. Available at: https://shop.elsevier.com/books/vascular-medicine-a-companion-to-braunwalds-heart-disease/creager/978-0-323-63600-1.

26. Neglen P, Raju S. A comparison between descending phlebography and duplex Doppler investigation in the evaluation of reflux in chronic venous insufficiency: a challenge to phlebography as the "gold standard". J Vasc Surg 1992;16(5):687–93.

27. Raju S, Knepper J, May C, et al. Ambulatory venous pressure, air plethysmography, and the role of calf venous pump in chronic venous disease. J Vasc Surg Venous Lymphat Disord 2019;7(3):428–40.

28. Gornik HL, Gerhard-Herman MD, Misra S, et al. Peripheral Vascular Ultrasound and Physiological Testing Part II: Testing for Venous Disease and Evaluation of Hemodialysis Access Technical Panel; Appropriate Use Criteria Task Force. ACCF/ACR/AIUM/ASE/IAC/SCAI/SCVS/SIR/SVM/SVS/SVU 2013 appropriate use criteria for peripheral vascular ultrasound and physiological testing part II: testing for venous disease and evaluation of hemodialysis access: a report of the american college of cardiology foundation appropriate use criteria task force. J Am Coll Cardiol 2013;62(7):649–65.

29. Locker T, Goodacre S, Sampson F, et al. Meta-analysis of plethysmography and rheography in the diagnosis of deep vein thrombosis. Emerg Med J 2006;23(8):630–5.

30. Bush R, Comerota A, Meissner M, et al. Recommendations for the medical management of chronic venous disease: The role of Micronized Purified Flavanoid Fraction (MPFF). Phlebology 2017;32(1_suppl):3–19 [Erratum in: Phlebology. 2017;32(10): NP36].
31. de Ávila Oliveira R, Riera R, Vasconcelos V, et al. Injection sclerotherapy for varicose veins. Cochrane Database Syst Rev 2021;12(12):CD001732.
32. Gohel MS, Heatley F, Liu X, et al, EVRA Trial Investigators. A Randomized Trial of Early Endovenous Ablation in Venous Ulceration. N Engl J Med 2018;378(22): 2105–14.
33. Barwell JR, Davies CE, Deacon J, et al. Comparison of surgery and compression with compression alone in chronic venous ulceration (ESCHAR study): randomised controlled trial. Lancet 2004;363(9424):1854–9.
34. Morrison N, Gibson K, McEnroe S, et al. Randomized trial comparing cyanoacrylate embolization and radiofrequency ablation for incompetent great saphenous veins (VeClose). J Vasc Surg 2015;61(4):985–94.
35. Lane T, Bootun R, Dharmarajah B, et al. A multi-centre randomised controlled trial comparing radiofrequency and mechanical occlusion chemically assisted ablation of varicose veins - Final results of the Venefit versus Clarivein for varicose veins trial. Phlebology 2017;32(2):89–98.

Lower-Extremity Vascular Ulcers

Assessment and Approaches to Management

James B. Alexander, MD, DFSVS

KEYWORDS

- Arterial ulcers • Leg ulcers • Lymphedema • Venous hypertension • Venous ulcers
- Leg wounds

KEY POINTS

- Chronic lower-extremity skin ulcers are often a complication of disorders of the arteries, veins, and/or lymphatics.
- Wound healing is the culmination of defined physiologic processes that can be negatively impacted by diseases and their treatments.
- Identifying specific causes of poor wound healing permits strategies to compensate for or eliminate obstacles to healing.

INTRODUCTION

Vascular leg ulcers are skin wounds of the lower extremities. They may occur de novo but are often the result of minor trauma that fails to heal normally. Their delayed healing is a consequence of underlying arterial, venous, and/or lymphatic disease. Their prevalence is difficult to determine but is likely in the range of 1% to 1.5%.[1,2] This figure varies depending on the age range being considered, as leg ulcers of all 3 varieties are more common with increasing age. This article will not specifically address leg ulcers associated with dermatologic causes, as these were addressed in a recent *Medical Clinics of North America* issue.[3] Vasculitic conditions are the subject of a separate article in this issue.

Arterial and venous leg ulcers are both caused by a derangement of regional hemodynamics. In arterial wounds, the regional arterial blood pressure is lower than normal at rest. In venous wounds, the regional venous blood pressure is higher than normal when the leg is dependent. However, venous hypertension may be ameliorated by elevating the leg above the heart, or even by activating the calf muscle pump with ambulation. The limb in arterial insufficiency withers while the limb in venous

Division Vascular Medicine, Jefferson Vascular Center, Sidney Kimmel Medical College, Thomas Jefferson University, 111 South 11th Street, Suite 6210, Philadelphia, PA 19107, USA
E-mail address: James.Alexander@jefferson.edu

Med Clin N Am 107 (2023) 911–923
https://doi.org/10.1016/j.mcna.2023.05.003
0025-7125/23/© 2023 Elsevier Inc. All rights reserved.

insufficiency swells. However, in neither condition does the circulation support normal wound healing.

Lymphatic wounds are included here for 2 reasons. First, the lymphatic system is rightly the third component of the vascular system. Second, derangement of lymphatic function is often concomitant of other vascular leg ulcers, especially venous leg ulcers. The lymphatic system does not convey whole blood, but it does participate in the clearing of fluid, metabolites, immune cells, and debris from the interstitial compartment of the periphery. Similar to the cause of venous leg ulcers, lymphatic dysfunction results from diminished flow away from the legs toward the central circulation, resulting in increased interstitial pressure and the accumulation of interstitial fluid.

ASSESSMENT
Arterial Ulcers

History
The diagnosis of arterial insufficiency is typically ascertained from a history of ischemic pain. Pain in relevant muscle groups with ambulation, or claudication, is evidence of ischemia with exercise. Whereas claudication is ischemia of muscles not skin, and then only with exertion, a lower-extremity skin ulcer that is not healing for lack of arterial perfusion implies resting ischemia. Other painful conditions of the lower extremities (eg, arthritis and neuropathy) need to be distinguished from arterial insufficiency.[4]

The pain associated with arterial insufficiency that impairs wound healing is typically in the most distal parts of the limb, in the feet or toes. It may be exacerbated at night when the feet are elevated in bed and may be relieved by getting the feet back into a dependent position. Such patients may find they sleep better sitting up in a chair than reclining flat. The resultant constant dependent position of the leg may result in lower-extremity swelling that mimics venous or lymphatic disease.

Physical examination
Physical examination of the leg with arterial insufficiency will usually reveal absent pedal pulses and sluggish capillary refill (>3 seconds). Nonetheless, the skin may look adequately perfused or, if the foot is dependent, even hyperemic (a finding known as dependent rubor). However, with elevation of the foot above the heart, pallor may be uncovered. Paradoxically, pedal pulses may be palpable in cases of distal atheroembolization (the blue toe syndrome).

Diagnostic studies
The diagnosis of arterial insufficiency is best confirmed by assessing local tissue perfusion. Imaging studies (duplex ultrasound, computed tomography [CT], MRI) yield anatomic information, but the diagnosis of ischemia is best supported by physiologic data. Ankle and toe pressures are readily measured in clinical vascular laboratories. Ankle pressures are generally more accurate but may be subject to systematic error in cases of noncompressible arteries (medial calcinosis) often found in patients with diabetes mellitus or end-stage renal disease. Toe pressures may be preferred in these patients because the digital vessels tend to remain compliant. Pressures may be indexed by dividing by patients' systemic systolic blood pressure, approximated by brachial systolic occlusion pressure.

Venous Ulcers

History
Venous leg ulcers are the most common and account for at least two-thirds of vascular leg ulcers.[5] Ambulatory venous hypertension may be the result of damage to lower-

extremity veins from trauma, surgery, and/or venous thrombosis, so a history should be obtained to elucidate these possibilities. A family history of venous thromboembolic disease may suggest an underlying genetic hypercoagulable condition. Venous hypertension may also occur de novo, as a result of venous valvular reflux, although there is often a family history of venous disease, suggesting a genetic cause. A family history of venous varicosities, leg swelling, hyperpigmentation at the ankles, and/or leg ulcers should be sought.

Physical examination
In the presence of profuse venous varicosities, the diagnosis of venous hypertension may seem obvious. However, ambulatory venous hypertension of a degree that impairs wound healing usually implies substantial pathologic condition in the deep venous system, which need not correlate with the presence of superficial varices. Hemosiderin deposition leading to hyperpigmentation around the ankle is characteristic of chronic venous hypertension. There may be scarring from previously healed leg ulcers around the ankles, and there may be sclerotic changes of the subcutaneous tissues of the ankles even in the absence of overt scars, referred to as lipodermatosclerosis or, in its most severe form, atrophie blanche.[6]

Edema of the subcutaneous tissues is characteristic of venous hypertension and is another important physical finding. The edema of venous hypertension typically spares the feet, because venous insufficiency leading to leg ulcers is usually driven by deep vein pathologic condition, and the venous drainage of the feet is predominantly into the superficial veins. Measurements of calf and ankle circumference permit quantification of the severity of edema and facilitate documenting patients' progress and response to treatment. Of course, if leg swelling and prominent veins are of recent onset, acute deep vein thrombosis may need to be excluded.

Obesity contributes to ambulatory venous hypertension. Negative intrathoracic pressure with inspiration helps draw venous blood up the inferior vena cava, but positive intrabdominal pressure resists venous blood flow into the inferior vena cava. Hence, as obesity increases, so do lower-extremity ambulatory venous pressures.[7]

Lower-extremity venous return is also driven by contraction of calf muscles, which compress the capacitance veins in the deep compartments of the leg. However, anything that compromises the function of the calf muscle pump (eg, paraplegia, stroke, neuropathy, ankle fusion) will exacerbate ambulatory venous hypertension and promote venous leg ulcers. Conversely, active contraction of the calf muscles, especially when the leg is dependent, will facilitate venous return and reduce venous blood pressures.

Diagnostic studies
Ambulatory venous hypertension is usually a clinical diagnosis. Both outflow obstruction and venous valvular reflux may contribute to venous hypertension, but despite ultrasound imaging, CT venogram, MR venogram, and contrast venography, imaging techniques do not correlate well with the severity of the clinical disease. Invasive measurement of pressures is possible, of course, but has been limited to research applications. Ambulatory venous plethysmography is an intriguing diagnostic modality but is not widely available in clinical practice.[8]

Lymphatic Ulcers

History
Lymphedema is diagnosed by a history of lower-extremity swelling. Swelling from primary lymphedema typically precedes any history of trauma, surgery, or infection. Its onset may be in childhood (typically adolescence) or as an adult. There may be a family history of lymphedema, suggesting a genetic contribution, but this is not essential.

Lymphedema may also develop secondary to events that may damage or compromise lymphatic drainage of the legs. Surgical procedures to remove groin and/or pelvic lymph nodes for cancer are the most obvious example. Similarly, radiation therapy to the groin or pelvic lymph nodes may cause sclerosis of lymphatic channels and result in lymphedema. Trauma, infection, or surgery of the lower extremity can damage lymphatic structure and function, resulting in chronic lymphedema. The accumulation and stasis of interstitial fluid in lymphedema predispose to cellulitis. Recurrent bouts of cellulitis can, in turn, further damage lower-extremity lymphatics, leading to a vicious cycle of increasing severity. The most common cause of acquired lymphedema worldwide is filariasis, but this is rare in North America.

Physical examination

Leg swelling may be symmetric, in which case systemic causes of lower-extremity swelling (cardiac, hepatic, or renal disease) may need to be explored. Asymmetric leg swelling, if acute, may of course warrant excluding deep vein thrombosis. Regional lymphadenopathy should also be evaluated and may be the first sign of underlying malignancy.

Lower-extremity swelling in lymphedema may include prominent involvement of the feet and even the toes (Stemmer sign). It is important to determine whether the swelling diminishes with leg elevation, typically overnight in bed. The Starling forces that drive the production of interstitial fluid in the subcutaneous tissues of the legs are substantially reduced if the feet are at the level of or above the heart. Therefore, if leg swelling does not diminish with elevation and the skin does not "pit" with digital compression, a diagnosis of lipedema should be considered. Lipedema also spares the foot, unlike lymphedema.

Diagnostic studies

The diagnosis of lymphedema is entirely clinical. Neither radiologic imaging nor physiologic assessment in the vascular laboratory is of help. Lymphangiograms were performed decades ago, when they were still used in the diagnosis and management of malignancies, but they are now rarely used in clinical practice. However, as surgeons continue to explore techniques for lymphatic reconstruction, methods of assessing lymphatic structure and function are being developed rapidly.[9]

Wound Assessment

History

Regardless of cause, wounds require specific assessment (**Box 1**). A history of how the wound started, how long it has been present, and how it has progressed or changed over time will provide clues to both the causes of the skin injury and the reason or reasons it is not healing. Also important is how the wound has been cared for. How has it been cleansed? What topical or systemic agents have been used to facilitate wound healing? How has it been dressed? How has it impacted the patient's activity or limited the patient? How painful is the wound, and how has the patient dealt with the pain? A history of fever or exudate from the wound will also guide management.

A complete medical and surgical history is important (**Table 1**). Special attention should be paid to conditions that may be associated with compromised wound healing (eg, diabetes mellitus, steroid use, immunosuppression in association with transplantation, cancer treatment, autoimmune diseases). In wounds of the lower extremities, conditions that may be associated with lower-extremity edema (eg, heart failure, renal failure, liver failure) or the use of diuretics (eg, hypertension) will be of interest. Also, a history of lower-extremity trauma and/or surgery may yield important

---

Box 1
Wound history

- How did the wound start?
- How long has it been there?
- How has it changed over time?
- How is it being cleansed?
- What topical agents have been applied?
- What systemic agents have been administered to aid healing?
- What dressings have been used, and how often are they changed?
- How much pain is associated with the wound?
- How much exudate is there from the wound?

---

clues, especially if there is prosthetic material retained in the affected limb. Although nutritional deficiencies are uncommon in North America, an inquiry into dietary habits, and sometimes a formal nutritional assessment, may be helpful.

Physical examination

Examination of wounds should include a detailed description of the location and size, including depth (**Box 2**). Color, texture (whether the skin is intact, partially preserved, or absent and its condition), the tissues/planes visible (subcutaneous fat, fascia, muscle, periosteum, bone, and so forth), any exudate, its character, and an estimate of its amount (scant, moderate, copious), and odor of wounds are all important. The peri-wound skin should be included in the examination (**Box 3**). Skin that is dry, cracked, hypertrophic, callused, macerated, indurated, or erythematous will have implications for management. The wound should be palpated, and tenderness, or conversely, the presence of neuropathy, should be assessed. Finally, if there is fluctance on palpation, there may be an indication for drainage of fluid, blood, or pus.

A diagnosis of invasive infection, cellulitis, or systemic sepsis is generally made on clinical grounds. Pronounced erythema of the peri–wound skin, swelling, and/or induration of the wound and peri–wound tissues, increased warmth of the periwound, and increased pain and tenderness of the wound are hallmarks of locally invasive infection. Systemic signs of fever, tachycardia, or hypotension suggest systemic sepsis.

Table 1
Medical/surgical history regarding vascular leg ulcer healing

• Conditions associated with compromised healing	• Diabetes mellitus
	• Autoimmune disease
	• Transplantation
	• Inflammatory conditions
	• Malignancy
• Conditions associated with leg swelling and/or diuretic use	• Heart failure
	• Hepatic disease
	• Hypertension
	• Lower-extremity cellulitis, surgery, or trauma
• Dermatologic diagnoses	• Renal insufficiency
• Diet/nutrition	• Venous thromboembolism

Box 2
Vascular leg ulcer physical characteristics

- Location
- Size (including depth)
- Color
- Texture (granular/slough/necrotic)
- Tissues exposed at base (subcutaneous fat, fascia, muscle, periosteum, bone)
- Exudate (character and quantity)
- Undermining
- Odor

Classification systems have been devised for wounds. A common classification designed for pressure injuries but used widely in clinical practice identifies 4 degrees of severity based on the level of wound penetration from the skin: (1) Damage to intact skin; (2) Partial-thickness skin loss; (3) Full-thickness skin penetration into subcutaneous fat; (4) Penetration to fascia, muscle, tendon, or bone[10] (**Box 4**).

A specific classification system has been developed for wounds in arterial insufficiency and is endorsed by the Society for Vascular Surgery known as the Wound, Ischemia, foot Infection (WIfI) risk stratification[11] (**Table 2**). This system incorporates a description of the degree of tissue injury, the physiologic severity of ischemia, and the presence or extent of infection. The WIfI score on initial presentation has been shown to correlate with the risk for leg amputation.[12]

Diagnostic studies

Initial wound assessment is usually limited to history and physical examination. Photographs, ideally with the inclusion of a ruler to allow calibration for measurements, are a useful adjunct to wound documentation and can facilitate monitoring progress. Further diagnostic studies may be directed at elucidating underlying vascular pathophysiology, as outlined above.

Microbiological cultures are rarely helpful and, therefore, are used selectively. Typically, if a clinical diagnosis of infection is made, empiric antibiotics will be indicated. Cultures may be confirmatory or allow focusing of antimicrobial therapy.

Wound biopsy is not typically helpful for the diagnosis of vascular leg ulcers per se, although it may be indicated to exclude other diagnoses. Biopsy may be indicated if a nonvascular cause is suspected, such as for an inflammatory vasculitis or dermatopathy.

Box 3
Periwound skin physical characteristics

- Moist/dry
- Intact/cracked/excoriated
- Hot/warm/cool
- Hypertrophic/callused/macerated/thin
- Indurated/edematous
- Erythematous/cyanotic/bruised

Box 4
Pressure injury staging system

- Stage 1: Intact skin with nonblanchable erythema
- Stage 2: Partial-thickness loss of skin with exposed, intact dermis
- Stage 3: Full-thickness loss of skin with extension into the subcutaneous adipose
- Stage 4: Full-thickness loss of skin with extension to fascia, muscle, tendon, ligament, cartilage, and/or bone

(Adapted from[10] with permission.)

In these instances, biopsy at the ulcer's edge, including some peri–wound skin, is usually the most helpful. Biopsy is also indicated if malignancy is suspected, in which case careful documentation of the biopsy site is mandatory to ensure its inclusion in subsequent extirpation, if indicated.

MANAGEMENT
Fundamentals

Wound healing is the conjunction of myriad metabolic and physiologic mechanisms inherent to human biology. There is no method or technique to make a wound heal. Optimal management permits wound healing to proceed unimpeded. Wound management is directed at identifying obstacles to normal wound healing and mitigating or overcoming those obstacles, thereby enabling wound healing.

The onset of a wound is the initial injury of the skin and/or subcutaneous tissues. Injury sets in motion the mechanisms to heal the wound. After hemostasis, the inflammatory phase is first. In simplest terms, the goal of the inflammatory phase of wound healing is to prepare the wound bed by removing debris and nonviable tissue and controlling bacterial contamination to prevent pathologic infection. Macrophages and polymorphonuclear leukocytes are prominent in the inflammatory phase. The inflammatory phase normally peaks in 24 hours and lasts about 3 days before starting to wane.[13]

Table 2
Wound, ischemia, foot infection classification system

Wound	0: No ulcer, no gangrene		
	1: Shallow ulcer (may have phalangeal exposure), no gangrene		
	2: Deep ulcer (exposed bone), gangrenous toe or toes		
	3: Deep ulcer, gangrene proximal to toes		
Ischemia		ABI	Ankle Pressure (mm Hg)	Toe Pressure (mm Hg)
	0	≥0.8	>100	≥60
	1	0.6–0.79	70–100	40–59
	2	0.4–0.59	50–70	30–39
	3	≤0.39	<50	<30
Foot infection	0: No infection		
	1: Local infection involving only skin & subcutaneous tissue		
	2: Local infection involving deep structures (abscess, osteomyelitis, septic arthritis, and similar)		
	3: Local infection with systemic signs		

(Adapted from[11] with permission.)

On about the third day following wounding, the proliferative phase begins. Collagen production and angiogenesis accelerate. Fibroblasts are prominent, although there appears to be a vital role for multipotential or stem cells, recruited from local tissues and/or bone marrow. The traditional marker of the progress of the proliferative phase has been the tensile strength of the wound (reflecting the production and organization of collagen). In normal wound healing, wound tensile strength is only 5% of the preinjury value after 1 week, 50% after 1 month, and 80% by 2 months.[13]

The third phase is wound maturation. During maturation, there is little change in tensile strength, but the volume of the wound, which now comprises scar tissue, diminishes. The scar will become flatter, softer, and paler. This is often associated with an improvement in cosmetic appearance, but the maturation process takes at least 6 months and often as much as a year. Nonetheless, even the fully healed wound/scar remains an active lesion indefinitely with increased collagen turnover. Hence, the finding that scars that have been healed for years spontaneously dehisce in scurvy (vitamin C deficiency).

On this background, then, it is important that a wound be clean and free of debris and foreign bodies. Gentle cleansing and copious lavage are useful. Harsh chemicals (hydrogen peroxide, isopropyl alcohol, iodine, sodium hypochlorite, and so forth) have little place. Mechanical debridement may be indicated.

The open wound is contaminated. Sterility is not an achievable goal outside of, perhaps, a formal operating room. Topical antimicrobials are touted for their ability to kill or suppress the growth of microorganisms. However, one might question whether the real issue is not what organisms they discourage, but rather which ones they allow, because those are the ones that will populate a wound following their application.

On the other hand, maintaining a moist environment is essential. Desiccation kills tissues at the wound surface, creating new, dead debris that requires removal for wound healing to progress. Topical ointments and foam or gel dressings are available to promote a moist, physiologically balanced wound environment while absorbing wound exudate and suppressing bacterial and/or fungal overgrowth. Periodic changing of these dressings will permit wound cleansing as well as renewal of a wound environment that will permit healing.[14]

An intact blister, with clear fluid and without excessive pain and/or erythema of adjacent tissues, may provide a suitable moist environment for a short time. However, it can easily become a nidus of infection and should be debrided before it does. Similarly, a firm, solidly adherent scab or eschar may be an effective barrier to protect the underlying tissues from desiccation or bacterial overgrowth while healing gets started but will require monitoring. Evidence of separation suggests the barrier is no longer effective, at which point the nonviable material should be carefully removed.[14]

Arterial Ulcers

The primary intervention for lower-extremity wounds that have a significant ischemic component is to restore adequate arterial flow. Both endovascular and open surgical techniques may be useful. Although moderate peripheral arterial disease (Ankle Brachial Index [ABI] >0.5) will often not interfere with healing, conditions that may compromise the microvasculature (eg, diabetes mellitus, radiation) often mandate the best arterial flow possible. When healing is thwarted by microvascular disease (radiation injury, diabetes mellitus) despite adequate arterial inflow, hyperbaric oxygen therapy may be a useful adjunct.

Care should be taken to avoid unduly compressive or constricting dressings in patients with arterial disease. Arterial blood flow is driven by blood pressure.

Compressive or constricting dressings may diminish blood flow, resulting in ischemia of the wound.

Although the removal of frankly dead or infected tissue is appropriate, debridement of ischemic wounds should be judicious. Specifically, debriding back to healthy, bleeding tissues should be avoided because in the face of ischemia the bleeding tissues that are injured will not heal and further tissue necrosis may ensue.

Infection of ischemic wounds is especially problematic. As already pointed out, bacterial colonization is common and of little clinical consequence. Correspondingly, antimicrobial therapy absent of clinical infection is of no utility. On the other hand, invasive infection is a risk of any open wound. Invasive infection warrants systemic antibiotics. However, in ischemic wounds, systemic antibiotics are unlikely to reach the wound sufficiently to be effective. Furthermore, even if the antibiotics could somehow be "forced" into the region of infection, absent of an influx of leukocytes and their ability to provide a vigorous oxidative attack on invading microbes, infection may still prevail.[15] Consequently, surgical consultation should be sought for infected ischemic wounds. Appropriate interventions may include drainage of abscess, debridement of nonviable tissues, and revascularization to alleviate the ischemia.

Venous Ulcers

The mainstay in the management of venous leg ulcers is compression therapy.[16] Compression is applied from the midfoot to the proximal calf, but short of the knee. Compression should be greater than 40 mm Hg.[17] Compression may be elastic or inelastic and may take the form of rolled dressings, stockings, or adjustable inelastic garments.[18]

High-grade compressive dressings require expertise to apply safely and effectively. They should be changed at least weekly, and more often if there is copious drainage from wounds. Healing often takes several months. Expedient healing is the goal, but on a week-by-week basis, it is sufficient to see progress with wounds granulating, becoming shallower, and closing in from the periphery.

Maintaining a clean ulcer bed is intuitive. Gentle cleansing with mild soap and water is fundamental. However, debridement and even surgical curettage may be used, although the benefits have not been well documented in the literature. The twin objectives are to remove slough and bioburden in order to achieve a clean ulcer bed, as well as to convert a stalled, chronic wound to an acute, healing wound by inciting a degree of inflammation (the first phase of wound healing). Debridement of venous leg ulcers is recommended by both the Society for Vascular Surgery and the American Venous Forum.[19]

Because both venous leg ulcers and peripheral arterial disease are more common with advancing age, it is not unusual to see patients in whom both are considerations. Moderate compression, greater than 40 mm Hg, may be applied if ankle pressure is greater than 60 mm Hg, toe pressure is greater than 30 mm Hg, and ABI is greater than 0.6. However, close monitoring of the patient is prudent, and compression should be abandoned if there is marked pain with compressive bandaging or if ulceration deteriorates. If arterial perfusion pressures are not adequate or compression is not tolerated, consideration should be given to arterial revascularization before using compression.[20]

Good skin hygiene is also fundamental to venous leg ulcer healing. A hypertrophic response of epidermal thickening and excessive dryness is common and is referred to as stasis eczema. This, in turn, can be associated with pruritis, which can result in scratching and excoriation, leading to additional skin injury. The use of hypoallergenic, nondrying soap for cleansing and liberal application of topical emollients will improve the skin texture, reduce epidermal hypertrophy, and ameliorate pruritis. Pharmacologic agents have also been identified to facilitate venous ulcer healing. They include flavonoids,[21] sulodexide,[22] and pentoxifylline,[23] but the evidence is of limited quality, and the improvement seen is modest.

Lymphatic Ulcers

The management of lymphatic ulcers parallels that of venous ulcers. In clinical practice, the two often overlap with coexistent pathologic condition of both vascular systems. The difference between them is that there are almost always more than sufficient veins for venous return, they simply are not working adequately when the leg is dependent. In severe lymphedema, there are often insufficient lymphatic channels to clear the accumulated interstitial fluid, so the emphasis is on limiting its accumulation in the first place.[24]

Elastic garments and stockings can be used for lymphedema management, but because the goal is to manipulate the Starling forces that drive interstitial fluid production, the pressures needed can be problematic. Inelastic garments that are applied when swelling has ebbed and that will not permit expansion of the subcutaneous compartment are often more easily used, better tolerated, and consequently more effective.[25]

Lymphedema pumps consist of leggings with multiple circumferential pneumatic compartments that are inflated sequentially to high pressures. These can also be crucial to the management of lymphedema. Although the pumps are only therapeutic for the hour or two a day that patients spend in them, their ability to achieve an acute reduction of subcutaneous interstitial fluid in the legs then permits the timely application of the garments described above that can maintain control of interstitial fluid accumulation.

Cleansing, debriding, and dressing lymphatic ulcers mirror the care of venous ulcers. Similarly, in lymphedema, the adjacent skin is subject to many of the same stresses as in ambulatory venous hypertension, so a clinical picture of stasis dermatitis is common. The use of hypoallergenic, nondrying soap for cleansing and liberal application of topical emollients will similarly improve and protect the skin.

PREVENTION OF RECURRENCE

The prevention of recurrent arterial ulcers is the maintenance of adequate arterial perfusion. This mandates the management of risk factors for atherosclerotic peripheral arterial occlusive disease. If the patient has undergone revascularization, by either endovascular techniques or open surgical intervention, then the maintenance of patency of those interventions, including both pharmacologic therapy and surveillance imaging, is crucial. However, the elaboration of these is beyond the scope of this article.

The recurrence rate of venous ulcers is high. Prevention of recurrence is similar to treatment, in that compression is key. However, compression is also unpopular, and once the ulcers are healed, patients' motivation can wane. Higher pressure is more effective in preventing recurrence, but lower pressure is better tolerated.[26,27] However, the lowest recurrence rates for venous leg ulcers correlate with the highest compliance in wearing compression garments, perhaps more than the degree of compression.[28]

The cause of venous leg ulcers is venous hypertension, often demonstrably the result of venous valvular reflux in the affected leg. Although deep venous reflux may be the primary driver, there is often a substantial component of superficial venous reflux. Studies have demonstrated lower recurrence rates following ablation of incompetent superficial veins, even in the presence of coexisting deep venous reflux.[29]

Furthermore, there may be an advantage to addressing superficial venous reflux to hasten the healing of extant venous ulcers.[30] Similarly, iliac and/or inferior vena caval obstruction (May-Thurner syndrome) may be alleviated by endovascular stenting with a reduction in venous leg ulcer recurrence.[31]

FAILURE TO HEAL

Everything in this article so far has focused on healing vascular leg ulcers. However, wound care practitioners recognize that some wounds do not heal—ever. However, this should be a designation that is only assigned after exhaustive attempts to heal the wound, and even then, the designation is only tentative. However, before deciding that a vascular leg ulcer will not heal, there are some things to consider.

Is the ulcer not healing, or is one ulcer healing yet another is appearing? The leg is never healed, but each individual ulcer may heal. This suggests an underlying skin disorder that is driving the development of new ulcers.

Is it fundamentally a skin disorder not caused by a vascular cause? Pyoderma gangrenosum, calciphylaxis, and skin cancers are examples of skin conditions that may be recalcitrant. Dermatologic conditions can coexist with arterial, venous, and/or lymphatic disease. In the event of a nonhealing leg ulcer, consultation with dermatology may help identify and curtail a cause, thereby permitting durable healing of the leg.

Is the patient manipulating the wound so as to prevent healing? The compressive dressings used for venous and lymphatic ulcers are often effective in preventing patients from getting access to their wounds, thereby allowing them to heal. Nonetheless, just as orthopedists are familiar with patients sliding objects inside their casts, patients may find a way to thwart the protection afforded by the compressive dressings. They may do it inadvertently, not realizing that they are undermining efforts to heal their ulcers, or they may do it for secondary gain.

Finally, if healing seems to evade all efforts, the best that may be achieved is stability and maintenance of the wound. Efforts should be directed at keeping the wound clean, keeping the wound free of infection, and minimizing its negative impact on the patient's quality of life. Chronic wounds are a burden, but effective wound care can help sustain the individual who must bear such a burden.

CLINICS CARE POINTS

- It is important to determine both the etiology of a leg ulcer and the factors that are impeding its healing.
- Cleansing a chronic wound to minimize devitalized tissue and reduce bioburden supports healing.
- Both desiccation and maceration of wounds slow healing. Wound dressings should be selected to maintain a moist environment but to avoid both desiccation and maceration.
- Venous leg ulcers are maintained by venous hypertension. Reduction of venous hypertension and compressive support are essential to achieve healing.
- Wounds complicated by ischemia require referral for revascularization.

DISCLOSURE

The author has nothing to disclose.

REFERENCES

1. Jawien A, Grzela T, Ochwatt A. Prevalence of chronic venous insufficiency in men and women in Poland: multicentre cross-sectional study of 40,095 patients. Phlebology 2003;18(3):110–22.
2. Rabe E, Pannier-Fischer F, Bromen K, et al. Bonner Venenstudie der deutschen gesellschaft fur phlebologieepidemiologische untersuchung zur frage der haufigkeit und auspragung von chronischen venekrankheiten in der stadtischen und landlichen wohnbevolkerung. Phlebology 2003;32(1):1–14.
3. Schneider CSS, Kirsner RS. Lower extremity ulcers. In: Callen J.P., Medical Clinics of North America. Elsevier; 2021. p. 663–79.
4. Conte MS, Bradbury AW, Kolh P, et al. Global vascular guidelines on the management of chronic limb-threatening ischemia. Eur J Vasc Endovasc Surg 2019; 58(1S):S1–109.
5. Tatsioni A, Balk E, O'Donnell TO, et al. Usual care in the management of chronic wounds: a review of the recent literature. J Am Coll Surg 2007;205(4):617–24.
6. Santler B, Goerge T. Chronic venous insufficiency-a review of pathophysiology, diagnosis, and treatment. J Dtsch Dermatol Ges 2017;15(5):538–56.
7. Willenberg T, Schumacher A, Amann-Vesti B, et al. Impact of obesity on venous hemodynamics of the lower limbs. J Vasc Surg 2010;52:664–8.
8. Raju S. Use of air plethysmography and ambulatory venous pressure measurement in chronic venous disease. Phlebolymphology 2020;27(2):52–60.
9. Watanabe S, Kajita H, Suzuki Y, et al. Photoacustic lymphangiography is a possible alternative for lymphedema staging. J Vasc Surg: Venous and Lymphatic Disorders 2022;10(6):1318–24.
10. Edsberg LE, Black JM, Goldberg M, et al. Revised national pressure ulcer advisory panel pressure injury staging system. J Wound Ostomy Continence Nurs 2016;43(6):585–97.
11. Mills JL, Conte MS, Armstrong DG, et al. The Society for Vascular Surgery lower extremity threatened limb classification system: risk stratification based on wound, ischemia, and foot infection (WIfI). Journal of Vascular Sugery 2014; 59(1):220–34.
12. Zhan LX, Branco BC, Armstrong DG, et al. The Society for Vascular Surgery lower extremity threatened limb classification system based on Wound, Ischemia, and foot Infection (WIfI) correlates with risk of major amputation and time to wound healing. J Vasc Surg 2015;61(4):939–44.
13. Martin P, Nunan R. Cellular and molecular mechanisms of repair in acute and chronic wound healing. Br J Dermatol 2015;173:370–8.
14. Rippon M, Davies P, White R. Taking the trauma out of wound care: the importance of undisturbed healing. J Wound Care 2012;(8):362, 364-368.
15. Lipsky BA, Berendt AR, Deery HG, et al. Diagnosis and treatment of diabetic foot infections. Plast Reconstr Surg 2006;117(7 Suppl):212S–38S.
16. O'Meara S, Cullum N, Nelson EA, Dumville JC. Compression for venous leg ulcers. Cochrane Database Syst Rev 2012;11(11):CD000265.
17. Milic DJ, Zivic SS, Bogdanovic DC, et al. The influence of different sub-bandage pressure values on venous leg uclers healing when treated with compression therapy. J Vasc Surg 2010;51(3):655–61.
18. Ashby RL, Gabe R, Ali S, et al. Clinical and cost-effectiveness of compression hoisery versus compression bandages in treatment of venous leg ulcers (Venous Leg Ulcer Study IV, VenUS IV): a randomised controlled trial. Lancet 2014;383: 871–9.

19. O'Donnell TF, Passman MA, Marston WA, et al. Management of venous leg ulcers: clinical practice guidelines of the Society for Vascular Surgery and the American Venous Forum. J Vasc Surg 2014;60(2S):3S–59S.
20. Humphreys ML, Stewart AH, Gohel MS, et al. Management of mixed arterial and venous leg ulcers. Br J Surg 2007;94:1104–7.
21. Scallon C, Bell-Syer SE, Aziz Z. Flavonoids for treating venous leg ulcers. Cochrane Database Syst Rev 2013;(5):CD006477.
22. Wu B, Lu J, Yang M, et al. Sulodexide for treating venous leg ulcers. Cochrane Database Syst Rev 2016;2016(6):CD010694.
23. Jull AB, Arroll B, Parag V, et al. Pentoxifylline for treating venous leg ulcers. Cochrane Database Syst Rev 2012;12(12):CD001733.
24. Burian EA, Karlsmark T, Norregaard S, et al. Wounds in chronic leg oedema. Int Wound J 2022;19(2):411–25.
25. Rabe E, Partsch H, Hafner J, et al. Indications for medical compression stockings in venous and lymphatic disease: an evidence-based consensus statement. Phlebology 2018;33(3):163–84.
26. Milic DJ, Zivic SS, Bogdanovic DC, et al. A randomized trial of class 2 and class 3 elastic compression in the prevention of recurrence of venous ulceration. J Vasc Surg: Venous and Lymphatic Disorders 2018;6(6):6717–23.
27. Kankam HKN, Lim CS, Fiorentino F, et al. A summation analysis of compliance and complications of compression hoisery for patients with chronic venous disease or post-thrombotic syndrome. Eur J Vasc Endovasc Surg 2018;55:406–16.
28. Clarke-Moloney M, Keane N, O'Connor V, et al. Randomised controlled trial comparing European standard class 1 to class 2 compression stockings for ulcer recurrence and patient compliance. Int Wound J 2014;11:404–8.
29. Gohel MS, Barwell JR, Taylor M, et al. Long term results of compression therapy alone versus compression plus surgery in chronic venous ulceration (ESCHAR): randomised controlled trial. Br Med J 2007;335:83–8.
30. Gohel MS, Heatley F, Liu X, et al. A randomized trial of early endovenous ablation in venous ulceration. N Engl J Med 2018;378(22):2105–14.
31. Yin M, Shi H, Ye K, et al. Clinical assessment of endovascular stenting compared with compression therapy alone in post-thrombotic patients with iliofemoral obstruction. Eur J Vasc Endovasc Surg 2015;50:101–7.

Vascular Imaging for the Primary Care Provider
Venous and Arterial Disease

Ammar A. Saati, MD[a], Craig Nielsen, MD[b],
Gerald Jay Bishop, MD[c],*

KEYWORDS

- Peripheral artery disease • Vasospastic disorders • Leg swelling
- Abdominal aortic aneurysm • Carotid artery disease • Vascular ultrasound

KEY POINTS

- This article will outline the clinical utility and value of the vascular lab in the diagnosis, treatment, and surveillance of common vascular diseases.
- Peripheral artery disease (PAD) is often underdiagnosed which can lead to significant cardiovascular morbidity and mortality. The vascular lab is instrumental in early detection of PAD as well as the ongoing surveillance of known disease, which can benefit in the selection of optimal therapies including medical management and interventions.
- Lower extremity swelling is a common complaint in primary care patients, and the vascular lab can help differentiate between the numerous underlying etiologies for this issue. DVT protocol or venous insufficiency studies help facilitate the diagnosis utilizing these non-invasive diagnostic modalities.
- Screening for abdominal aortic aneurysms (AAA) is an important part of general health maintenance and can be accomplished using arterial duplex ultrasound. This imaging technique can also be utilized for expansion surveillance in patients with a known AAA, using consensus guidelines for imaging intervals.
- Carotid artery disease can be diagnosed and followed on a serial basis utilizing carotid artery duplex ultrasound. Screening for carotid artery disease is not recommended for asymptomatic patients.

APPROACH TO THE SUSPECTED PERIPHERAL ARTERY DISEASE PATIENT

Peripheral artery disease (PAD) most often describes lower extremity obstructive arterial disease with the most common etiology of atherosclerosis. PAD affects approximately 8 to 12,000,000 people in the US and over 200 million people worldwide.

[a] Section of Vascular Medicine, Cleveland Clinic, 9500 Euclid Avenue, J 3-5, Cleveland, OH 44195, USA; [b] Internal Medicine and Geriatrics, Department of Internal Medicine, Cleveland Clinic, 9500 Euclid Avenue, G10, Cleveland, OH 44195, USA; [c] Section of Vascular Medicine, Cleveland Clinic, J 3-5, Cleveland, OH, USA
* Corresponding author.
E-mail address: bishopg@ccf.org

Med Clin N Am 107 (2023) 925–943
https://doi.org/10.1016/j.mcna.2023.05.004
medical.theclinics.com

The incidence increases with age and the prevalence is nearly twice as high in the African American population as compared to the Caucasian population. PAD affects men and women equally, and is a strong predictor of mortality, myocardial infarction, and stroke. Risk factors for PAD include age, hypertension, hyperlipidemia, diabetes, advanced chronic kidney disease, tobacco use, and a genetic disposition. Unfortunately, PAD is often under diagnosed and undertreated, and this can lead to excessive morbidity or mortality. The diagnosis of PAD should be entertained in patients at high risk or who have clinical features suggestive of this disease. This can be challenging as the majority of patients can be asymptomatic. The minority of patients will relate classic symptoms of intermittent claudication or present with ischemic rest pain. Consideration for PAD is recommended in patients with symptoms of claudication, atypical leg pain, functional impairment, significant cardiovascular risk factors, abnormal lower extremity pulse exam, non-healing wounds, or ischemic rest pain.[1–5]

Patients with risk factors and clinical features suggestive of peripheral artery disease should undergo a comprehensive vascular evaluation. Physical examination should include bilateral brachial artery blood pressures, skin examination, and examination of peripheral arteries including palpation and auscultation. Patients with PAD have an increased risk of subclavian artery stenosis and should have bilateral brachial blood pressures obtained at the initial encounter. Pressure gradients greater than 15 to 20 mm Hg are abnormal and suggestive of subclavian (or innominate) stenosis. Skin changes in PAD include mottling, arterial ulcers, gangrene, limb or digital color changes, or coolness to touch. Peripheral pulses should be examined including auscultation for bruits, and palpation of femoral, popliteal, and distal pulses including the dorsalis pedal and posterior tibial artery.

Diagnostic imaging involves the vascular lab and guidelines for imaging include surveillance for patients with established vascular disease, post intervention or surgery imaging, at-risk individuals (age > 65, age 50–64 with risk factors for atherosclerosis, age <50 with diabetes + 1or more risk factor for atherosclerosis, patient with non-healing wound and ulcers) and in patients with suspected PAD based on history and physical examination findings listed above.

Functional assessment includes the ankle and toe brachial index, exercise ankle brachial index (ABI), and pulse volume recordings (PVRs).[6] The ABI can be easily utilized in the office setting to diagnose PAD. Blood pressure cuffs are placed on the upper arms and ankles bilaterally and inflated above systolic pressure. As the pressure is released, the onset of flow is detected by the placement of a Doppler probe over the brachial and both pedal arteries (posterior tibial and dorsalis pedis). The ABI of each leg is calculated by dividing the higher of the two pedal arteries by the higher of the arm blood pressure. An ABI of less than 0.9 is used to make the diagnosis of PAD. The ABI has a sensitivity of 68% to 84% and a specificity of 84% to 99% for the diagnosis of PAD. Limitations of the ABI include medial arterial calcification resulting in non-compressible arteries that may lead to false elevation (ABI > 1.4) or artificial normalization of ABI. The ABI may also be normal or borderline abnormal at rest in patients with aortoiliac disease Interpretation of PAD is based on numerical findings as outlined in **Table 1**.[7] **Fig. 1** depicts the technical aspects of obtaining an ankle brachial index.

Exercise ABI may be helpful in unmasking PAD (especially proximal aorta iliac inflow disease) with normal resting ABI's. Patients with PAD may be asymptomatic at rest and only develop claudication symptoms with exertion. In such individuals, it is possible for resting ABI measurements to be normal. As a result, when the suspicion for PAD is high and resting measurements are normal, it is recommended to obtain an exercise ABI. Usual protocols involve fixed treadmill settings of 2 miles per hour at a 2% grade for a maximum of 5 minutes. Pre- and post-exercise ABI can be obtained

Table 1
Interpretation of ankle-brachial index (ABI)

Ankle-Branchial Index (ABI)	Interpretation
1.0–1.4	Normal
0.91–0.99	Borderline range
0.70–0.90	Mildly abnormal
0.40–0.69	Moderately abnormal
<0.40	Severely abnormal
>1.4	Incompressible vessels

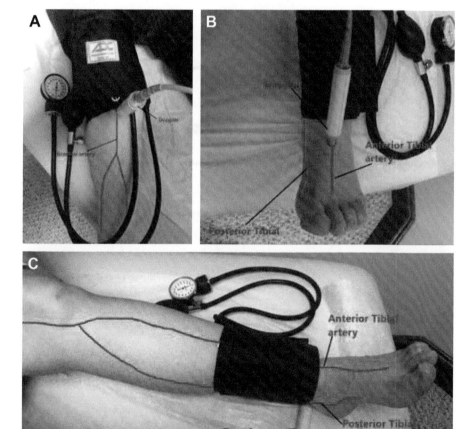

Fig. 1. Performing an ABI. (*A*) Measurement of blood pressure at the level of brachial artery. (*B*) Pulse volume recording at the area of anterior tibial artery and posterior tibial artery by doppler ultrasound. (*C*) Measurement of blood pressure at the level of lower leg. (Photographs courtesy of G. Jay Bishop M.D.)

with an abnormal result defined as a decrease in the post exercise ankle pressures and/or ABI result by greater than 20%. Claudication symptoms can be reproduced with exercise and quantified regarding time and distance as well. **Fig. 2** depicts an abnormal exercise ABI study with a drop in ankle pressures and ABI greater than 20%, consistent with exercise induced peripheral artery disease.

Pulse volume recording (PVR) is a non-invasive physiologic imaging modality that is helpful in the care of the patient with suspected or known PAD. This test refers to the graphic representation of the change in volume of the pulse contour in a specific segment of the extremity during the cardiac cycle. They are typically obtained by using BP cuffs placed at the high thigh, low thigh, calf, ankle, midfoot, and toe and may be used in

Lower Arterial Exercise Pressures

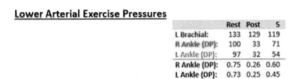

	Rest	Post	S
L Brachial:	133	129	119
R Ankle (DP):	100	33	71
L Ankle (DP):	97	32	54
R Ankle (DP):	0.75	0.26	0.60
L Ankle (DP):	0.73	0.25	0.45

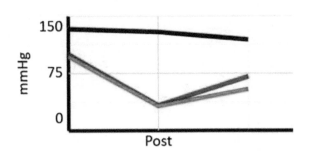

Lower Arterial Exercise Waveforms

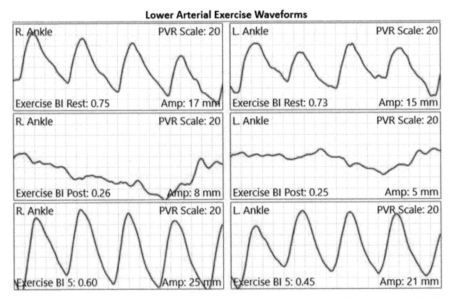

Fig. 2. Exercise ankle brachial index study – pre- and post- Exercise. Ankle pressure and ABI. (Images courtesy of Cleveland Clinic Foundation Vascular Lab.)

conjunction with segmental pressures. PVRs are usually paired with the ABI as a single test at most vascular labs as PVR can help localize anatomic segments of the disease (in contrast to the ABI). PVRs also have the advantage in patients with noncompressible vessels as they can still yield diagnostic information through review of the pulse volume contours and amplitude. They also can localize diseases including aorta iliac inflow, femoral/popliteal, infrapopliteal, and small vessel disease. However, despite their ability to localize disease, PVR measurements do not yield any information about specific lesion characteristics (ie, length, occlusion) and have decreased sensitivity for distal disease when inflow disease is present. Abnormal PVR findings include decreased amplitude, flattened peaks, absent dicrotic notch, and decreases in segmental pressure gradients between cuffs greater than 20 mm Hg which aid in the diagnosis of arterial occlusive disease. Examples of a normal PVR study are noted in **Fig. 3**.

Anatomic assessment can be obtained utilizing *arterial duplex ultrasound*. This noninvasive modality is a useful adjunct to non-invasive physiologic testing. This test is typically obtained for a more focused evaluation of the lower extremity arterial system. This imaging option utilizes a combination of B-mode ultrasound (US) imaging and spectral Doppler analysis. Doppler complements the standard qualitative US imaging by allowing waveform analysis and assessment of peak systolic velocities (PSV). Using the concept that the velocity of blood flow increases as it flows through a stenotic lesion, peak systolic and end-diastolic velocities are measured and used to estimate the severity of stenosis. Arterial flow characteristics can be normal or abnormal.

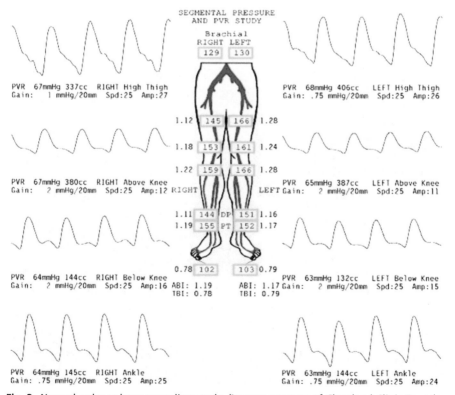

Fig. 3. Normal pulse volume recording study. (Images courtesy of Cleveland Clinic Foundation Vascular Lab.)

This modality is useful for the anatomic visualization of lesions and for surveillance after stenting or bypass grafting. Arterial duplex ultrasonography can indicate the level and severity of occlusions, patency of stents or bypass grafts, evaluate AV fistulas for dialysis, and screen for pseudoaneurysms and other post-interventional or post-surgical complications. A class IIa recommendation is given for routine surveillance using duplex ultrasound following infrainguinal revascularization with a goal of early identification of high-grade stenosis (PSV > 300 cm/s) and impending graft failure (PSV < 40 cm/s).[7] Duplex image of normal flow through the right superficial femoral artery is noted in **Fig. 4**. **Table 2** outlines the diagnostic criteria for PAD utilizing peak systolic velocities and velocity ratios. These velocity criteria are less reliable when interrogating the infra-popliteal arteries.[8] **Fig. 5** depicts arterial duplex ultrasonography of a patent popliteal stent with gray scale and color flow images.

The approach to the patient suspected of peripheral artery disease includes utilization of the vascular lab for optimal diagnostic value. **Fig. 6** provides guidance on the diagnostic approach to the patient with suspected PAD. AHA/ACC consensus guidelines give a Class I recommendation for patients with history or physical examination finding suggestive of PAD, the resting ABI, with or without segmental pressures and waveforms is recommended to establish the diagnosis. A IIa recommendation is given in patients at increased risk of PAD but without history or physical examination finding suggestive or PAD, measurement of resting ABI is reasonable.[9]

APPROACH TO THE SUSPECTED VASOSPASTIC DISORDER

Vasospastic disorders are conditions that occur when blood flow is disturbed related to arterial or arteriolar spasms. This can result in mild color changes to severe ischemic pain and necrotic changes. This can involve several vascular conditions,

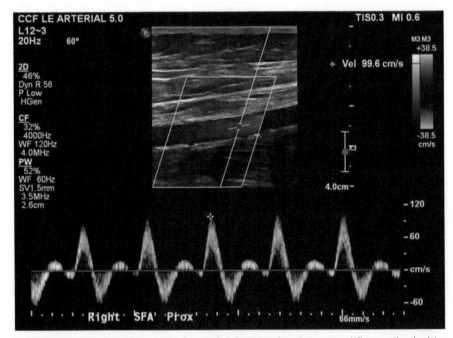

Fig. 4. Duplex arterial ultrasound of superficial artery showing normal flow and velocities. (Images courtesy of Cleveland Clinic Foundation Vascular Lab.)

Table 2
Diagnostic criterial for lower extremity arterial duplex scan for peripheral arterial disease (PAD)

Degree of Stenosis	Peak Systolic Velocity (cm/s)	Velocity Ratio
<20%	<150	<1.5
20%–49%	150–200	1.5–2.0
50%–80%	200–300	2.0–4.0
>80%	>300	>4.0
Occlusion	No flow detected in lumen	N/A

Adapted from Hodgkiss-Harlow KD & Bandyk DF. Semin Vasc Surg 2013;95-104.

including Raynaud's phenomena (that can be primary or secondary), acrocyanosis, peripheral cyanosis, pernio, and erythromelalgia.[10] Comprehensive history, physical examination and vascular laboratory testing are necessary to identify and assess the underlying etiology.

Raynaud's is caused by dysregulated constriction of the precapillary arterioles that lead to changes in skin color, swelling, and paresthesia. It generally affects the fingers and toes but can also affect other sites such as the nose, ears, and nipples.[11] Furthermore, Acrocyanosis is due to a decrease in the amount of oxygen delivered to the tissues of the extremities, and the precise mechanism remains elusive. Potential pathophysiological disturbances include abnormal arteriolar tone, alteration of microvascular responsiveness with capillary and venular dilation and stasis, and abnormal sympathetic nervous activity.[12] In contrast to Raynaud's, the bluish discoloration of acrocyanosis is persistent rather than episodic and is not associated with discomfort.

Noninvasive vascular laboratory testing can be used to document the presence and severity of vasospasm, assess for improvement with warming, establish an individual patient baseline and monitor improvement with therapy. Digital waveforms and thermal provocation studies are integral strategies in the approach to the patient with a suspected vasospastic disorder. Extremity segmental pressures include digital systolic pressures, sometimes with a temperature challenge. Digital waveforms can be mild, moderate dampening, or severely abnormal with flattening waveform. The measurement of cold recovery time is a classic test that utilizes photoplethysmography (PPG) or laser Doppler to monitor digital blood flow. Pulse volume recording can

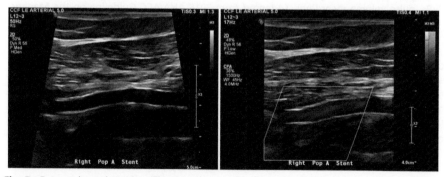

Fig. 5. Gray scale and Duplex ultrasound imaging of patent popliteal artery stent. (Images courtesy of Cleveland Clinic Foundation Vascular Lab.)

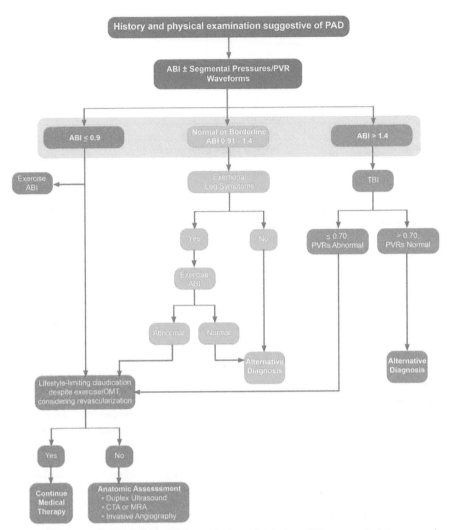

Fig. 6. Diagnostic pathway PAD. ABI, ankle-brachial index; CTA, computed tomography angiography; MRA, magnetic resonance angiography; PAD, peripheral artery disease; PVRs, pulse volume recordings. (*Adapted from* 2016 AHA/ACC Guideline on the Management of Patients with Lower Extremity Peripheral Artery Disease.)

detect severe small vessel disease, fixed occlusive disease, ischemia, and/or vaso-spasm. PPG waveforms can be normal, reduced, or absent pulsatility. Doppler flow studies with a thermal challenge can be employed to evaluate pathologic response to heat or cold. Thermal provocation with warming is usually preferred to minimize patient discomfort if baseline digital waveforms are abnormal. **Fig. 7** provides guidance on the diagnostic approach for vasospastic disorder.

The purpose of the vascular lab in evaluating the upper extremities to identify, localize and quantify obstruction of the arteries supplying the circulation to the arms and fingers. This may not be offered in all vascular labs. The basic procedural protocol includes placing blood pressure cuffs on the upper or lower extremity and the middle

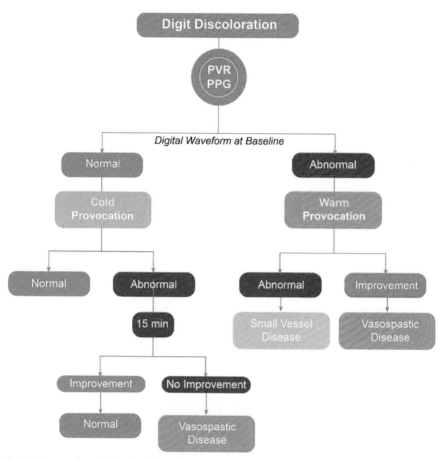

Fig. 7. Approach to digit discoloration.

digit at the base. Digital waveforms can be taken with a PPG sensor taped to the tip of fingers. Doppler waveforms are recorded in bilateral radial and ulnar arteries.[13] **Fig. 8** depicts an abnormal PPG recording with significant improvement after warming provocation.

APPROACH TO THE SWOLLEN LEG

Lower extremity swelling is a common presentation for primary care providers and the emergency department. Identification of the underlying etiology can be challenging but is important, as limb swelling may have a significant impact on the patient. Lower extremity swelling is usually a result of an increase in the interstitial fluid that exceeds the physiologic capacity of lymphatic absorption and drainage.[14] The swelling can be acute or chronic, as well as primary or secondary. A practical diagnostic approach to efficiently identify the causes of swelling includes a complete history and physical examination, and appropriate vascular ultrasound laboratory testing. The basic ultrasound examination for vascular and non-vascular etiologies is low cost and non-invasive. The vascular lab is helpful in evaluating the deep and superficial lower

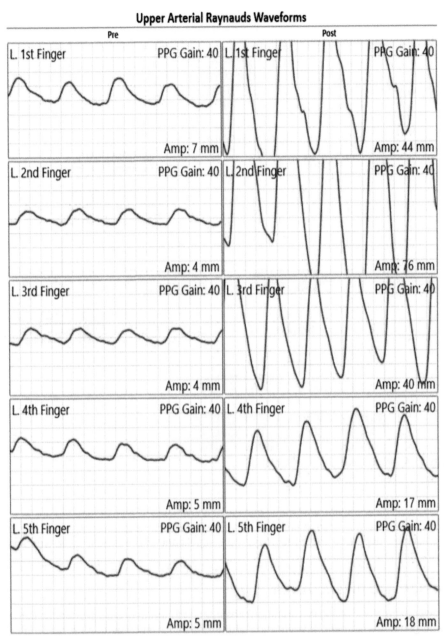

Fig. 8. Photoplethysmogram (PPG) tracing with improvement with warming provocation. (Images courtesy of Cleveland Clinic Foundation Vascular Lab.)

extremity venous system for the presence of thrombosis, reflux, or even suggestive evidence for more proximal stenosis or high systemic venous pressure by waveform abnormalities. Additional vascular ultrasound images can be obtained, particularly the Inferior Vena Cava (IVC), and common iliac veins, assessing unusual vessel sites like the visceral vessels by recording patency of the vessels by color and waveform Doppler. Dedicated venous insufficiency studies allow evaluation for venous incompetency in both deep and superficial veins, along with perforator veins and varicose veins if present. When encountering masses or cysts adjacent to the vessels, more detailed images are acquired, obtaining the size, and describing the consistency, in addition to the presence of vascularity by color Doppler. Documenting the presence of subcutaneous edema is usually not required but possibly mentioned in the final ultrasound report.

DVT protocol duplex venous ultrasound determines the presence or absence of thrombosis in the veins of the legs, identifies the exact location and extent of any identified thrombus and allows qualitative analysis of its characteristics. Acute DVT is characterized by a dilated vein, the presence of intraluminal echoes (usually echo lucent), and thrombus characteristics include spongy, organized, and poorly attached to the vein wall. The inability to coapt the walls of the vessel on compression maneuvers with the ultrasound probe is the most important aspect of diagnosing acute DVT. In contrast with non-acute and chronic DVT, the thrombus appears more echogenic, has a rigid texture, and is more attached to the walls. Other echotexture and acoustic properties include irregular borders, focal venous wall thickening, large collateral veins, normal or atrophic size veins, the presence of reflux, and recanalization of prior DVT. When assessing for thrombus, interrogation of the superficial veins and evaluating for superficial vein thrombophlebitis is an integral part of the imaging study. **Fig. 9** depicts an abnormal compression for the femoral vein indicating a noncompressible vein and a deep vein thrombosis.

When assessing for suspected venous insufficiency, a specific venous duplex test must be ordered, commonly known as a venous insufficiency or venous reflux study.

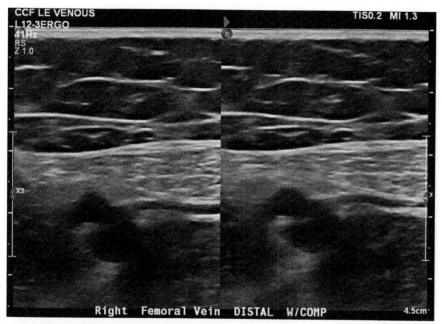

Fig. 9. Abnormal compression of the femoral vein indicating an acute DVT. (Images courtesy of Cleveland Clinic Foundation Vascular Lab.)

This duplex imaging of the extremity is performed to assess the deep and superficial venous system for the presence of deep or superficial venous incompetence and to document the location and severity of disease. These are time consuming and labor-intensive studies and should usually be ordered based on specific symptoms of leg heaviness, aching, swelling, throbbing, or itching, also known by the mnemonic HASTI. It is advisable only to interrogate the affected limb; these tests are usually ordered when contemplating any potential role for venous intervention. Positive findings of valvular incompetency are defined as retrograde (reflux) venous flow with Valsalva or augmentation maneuvers with durations of greater than 1 second for deep veins and greater than 0.5 seconds for superficial veins. Negative valvular incompetency demonstrates no retrograde venous flow with Valsalva and augmentation maneuvers or retrograde flow of less than 1 second of deep veins or less than 0.5 seconds of superficial veins. **Fig. 10** depicts a venous insufficiency study of the small saphenous vein with abnormal reflux greater than 0.5 seconds.[15] Air plethysmography (APG) is another tool to evaluate for venous insufficiency. APG is a non-invasive test that measures venous hemodynamics that quantify volume changes in the lower extremity with certain techniques.[16] Although APG has been clinically validated it is not widely used and not available in all vascular laboratories.

APPROACH TO ABDOMINAL AORTIC ANEURYSM AND CAROTID ARTERY STENOSIS

Abdominal aortic aneurysms (AAA) and Carotid artery Stenosis (CAS) are two common conditions primary care physicians will see in their clinical practice. The vascular lab plays an integral part in the care of patients with these vascular disorders, specifically with the appropriate use of aorta and carotid artery duplex ultrasound. We briefly outline screening recommendations, disease monitoring recommendations and the importance of risk factor modification in these patients.

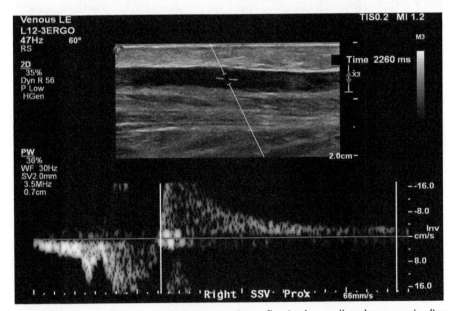

Fig. 10. Venous insufficiency study demonstrating reflux in the small saphenous vein. (Images courtesy of Cleveland Clinic Foundation Vascular Lab.)

ABDOMINAL AORTIC ANEURYSMS (AAA)
Screening

Abdominal aortic aneurysms (AAA) are typically defined as aortic enlargement greater or equal to 3 cm in diameter. AAAs are often asymptomatic and are found through screening, incidentally on imaging done for other indications, or at the time of rupture. Since they are often asymptomatic, screening high-risk populations is deemed an evidence-based approach to find AAA earlier in the disease course. In 2019, the United States Preventive Services Task Force (USPSTF) updated their recommendations for AAA screening.[17]

- B recommendation (moderate net benefit) - For men aged 65 to 75 who have ever smoked, it is recommended to perform a one-time screening for AAA with ultrasonography
- C recommendation (small net benefit) – For men aged 65 to 75 who have never smoked, screening for AAA can be recommended selectively based on the patients' medical and family history, risk factors and patients' preferences/values.
- D recommendation (potential harms > benefits) - Do not screen women aged 65 to 75 who have never smoked.
- I recommendation (insufficient evidence) - the evidence for screening in women aged 65 who have smoked is currently insufficient to determine net benefit.

The 2022 American College of Cardiology/American Heart Association (ACC/AHA) Aortic Disease guidelines differ slightly from USPSTF guidelines.[18] The ACC/AHA guidelines recommend AAA ultrasound screening in men > to 65 years of age who have ever smoked and in men or women who are greater than 65 years of age and who are first-degree relatives of patients with AAA (Strength of Recommendation – Strong, Class 1). In addition, they state it is reasonable to consider ultrasound screening in women greater than 65 years of age who have ever smoked. (Moderate, Class 2a recommendation) The guidelines also state that one could consider ultrasound screening in men or women less than age 65 if they have multiple risk factors or a strong family history of AAA. (Weak, Class 2b recommendation) Lastly, the guideline states that there is no benefit to repeating ultrasound screening in men or women greater than 75 years of age who are asymptomatic and have had a negative initial ultrasound screen.

The 2018 Society of Vascular Surgery (SVS) guidelines call for a one-time screening ultrasound in all men and women aged 65 to 75 with the history of tobacco use (Level 1 recommendation, quality of evidence High). (19) In addition, the SVS states that ultrasound screening for AAA in patients who have first degree relatives with an AAA should be considered. (Level 2 recommendation, quality of evidence low).

In summary, The USPSTF, ACC/AHA and SVS all agree that it is appropriate to screen men age greater than 65 who have smoked. The ACC/AHA and SVS guidelines also include women who have smoked and patients with a strong family history of AAA in their screening recommendations.

Abdominal aortic aneurysms are also identified incidentally on imaging done for other indications, whether this be computed tomography (CT) studies, ultrasound studies, or magnetic resonance imaging (MRI) studies. The prevalence rate of incidental AAA has been estimated at 1% to 2%.[19,20] There is some data to suggest that incidentally found AAAs are often not monitored appropriately during follow up.[19] Appropriate protocols should be in place when AAAs are found incidentally to alert the ordering physician or primary care physician about the need for follow up.

Surveillance

Once discovered, it is important to follow surveillance guidelines to monitor AAA expansion. Repairs are usually recommended when an AAA is greater than 5.5 cm or for aneurysms that have expanded greater than 1 cm in a year. The interval between screening tests is determined by the size of the initial aneurysm. The ACC/AHA guidelines recommend the following monitoring intervals.[18]

Male Patients

- 3 to 3.9 cm in diameter: Ultrasound (US) every 3 years (Strong, Class 1 recommendation)
- 4 to 4.9 cm in diameter: US every 12 months (Strong, Class 1 recommendation)
- Greater than 5.0 cm in diameter: US every 6 months (Strong, Class 1 recommendation)

Female Patients

- 3 to 3.9 cm in diameter: Ultrasound (US) every 3 years (Strong, Class 1 recommendation)
- 4 to 4.4 cm in diameter: US every 12 months (Strong, Class 1 recommendation)
- Greater than 4.5 cm in diameter: US every 6 months (Strong, Class 1 recommendation)

If ultrasound images are suboptimal (eg, secondary to body habitus), then surveillance CT is recommended.

The Society of Vascular Surgery Guidelines recommend the following monitoring intervals for both male and female patients.[21]

- 3.0 to 3.9 cm in diameter – US every 3 years (level of recommendation – Weak; quality of evidence – low)
- 4.0 to 4.9 cm in diameter – US every year (level of recommendation – Weak; quality of evidence – low)
- 5.0 to 5.4 cm in diameter – US every 6 months (level of recommendation – Weak; quality of evidence – low)

The SVS recommends a referral to a vascular surgeon at the time of the initial diagnosis of an aortic aneurysm. They also recommend consideration of an elective repair once the AAA is > 5.5. cm in men and between 5.0 and 5.4 cm in women. (19) **Fig. 11** depicts an infrarenal abdominal aortic aneurysm measuring 5.04 cm in the transverse view.

Risk Factor Modification

Risk factors for abdominal aortic aneurysm are similar in scope to risk factors for coronary artery disease. Strong risk factors include smoking history, older age, male sex, and a positive family history of AAA. (18) Additional risk factors include hypertension, hyperlipidemia, white race, inherited vascular connective tissue disorder and atherosclerotic cardiovascular disease.[18] Although outcome data is limited regarding medical management/risk factor modification on AAA disease progression, the primary care physician should focus on helping the patient control modifiable risk factors (such as smoking, hypertension, and hyperlipidemia), which will also improve overall cardiovascular health. The ACC/AHA guidelines recommend antihypertensive medication in patients with AAA who have an average systolic blood pressure greater than 130 mm Hg or an average diastolic blood pressure greater than 80 mm Hg. (Strong, Class 1 recommendation).[18] The SVS guidelines does not recommend administering beta-blocker therapy for the sole purpose of reducing the risk of AAA expansion and rupture (Level

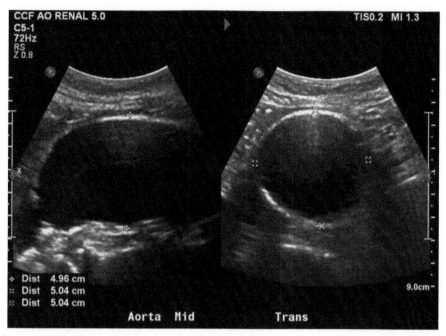

Fig. 11. Abdominal Aortic Aneurysm measuring 5.04 cm.in transverse diameter. (Images courtesy of Cleveland Clinic Foundation Vascular Lab.)

of recommendation – Strong, Quality of evidence – moderate).[21] In patients with AAA who have evidence of aortic atherosclerosis, the ACC/AHA guidelines recommend moderate to high intensity statin therapy. (Strong, Class 1 recommendation).[18] Smoking sensation is recommended in all patients with AAA.

APPROACH TO CAROTID ARTERY STENOSIS (CAS)
Screening

The USPSTF and SVS guidelines do not recommend screening for asymptomatic carotid stenosis in the general population.[22,23]

- USPSTF – Recommends against screening for asymptomatic carotid stenosis in the general population. (D recommendation)
- SVS – recommends against screening in asymptomatic patients without symptoms or significant risk factors for carotid disease (Grade 1(strong); quality of evidence: B (moderate))

The SVS guidelines state that screening in asymptomatic patients at increased risk for carotid stenosis should be considered, particularly in patients willing to consider intervention if significant stenosis is found. (Grade 2(weak); quality of evidence: B (moderate)).[23] This high-risk group includes patients with peripheral artery disease, coronary artery disease, previous radiotherapy to the neck and patients with evidence of previous cerebral infraction on brain imaging. The presence of a carotid bruit on physical exam is a common indication for testing. However, the presence of severe carotid disease in patients with a bruit and no other risk factors is only 2%.[22–26] The recommended screening test is a carotid artery duplex ultrasound performed in an accredited vascular lab. **Fig. 12** depicts right internal carotid artery stenosis.

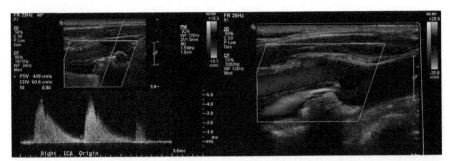

Fig. 12. Carotid Artery Stenosis right internal carotid artery with elevated peak systolic velocities. (Images courtesy of Cleveland Clinic Foundation Vascular Lab.)

Surveillance

Once carotid artery stenosis is diagnosed, a common question arises about the frequency of follow-up ultrasound examinations to document disease progression. Strong evidence-based guidelines to answer this question are lacking and recommendations are based on expert opinion. Patients found to have moderate stenosis (50% to 79%) should be followed up initially at 6-month intervals to detect disease progression that may require intervention.[27] Patients with less than 50% carotid stenosis can be followed initially annually.[27] Patients with severe stenosis (>79%) should be referred to a vascular specialist for further evaluation and management.

Risk Factor Modification

All patients diagnosed with carotid artery stenosis should be evaluated and treated with risk factor modification. Medical therapy has narrowed the gap between the medical and surgical treatment of carotid artery disease in reducing the risk of stroke. In patients with carotid artery stenosis, the annual risk of ipsilateral stroke is estimated to be 0.5%.[28] Moderate carotid artery stenosis is often more closely associated with myocardial infarction than stroke.[29] The core components of risk factor modification include lifestyle modification (eg, diet, exercise), blood pressure control, intensive lipid lowering, Diabetic control, B vitamin supplementation in patients with elevated homocysteine levels and smoking cessation.[28,30,31]

CLINICS CARE POINTS

- The best screening tool for peripheral artery disease (PAD) is the ankle brachial index (ABI).
- The PVR (pulse volume recording with segmental pressures) study is another first line study in the suspected PAD patient. Lower arterial duplex examinations are usually reserved for anatomical identification of known disease and surveillance of arterial interventions.
- If the ABI is normal and suspicion for PAD is still present, an exercise ABI can be helpful to unmask PAD.
- PAD is not just a leg disease, but a brain and heart disease as well given the association with stroke and MI.
- The mnemonic for venous insufficiency symptoms is HASTI (heaviness, aching, swelling, throbbing, and itching).
- Venous duplex ultrasound available for the legs include DVT protocol and a more complete venous insufficiency study.

- Surveillance regimens for AAA and carotid artery disease are important strategies in patients with known vascular pathology to document stability or progression.

- Patient history, examination, as well as the vascular lab can be helpful in diagnosis thermally provoked vasospastic disease such as Raynaud's.

DISCLOSURE

The authors have no significant commercial or financial disclosures relative to this manuscript submission.

REFERENCES

1. Criqui MH, Aboyans V. Epidemiology of peripheral artery disease. Circ Res 2015; 116(9):1509–26.
2. Fowkes FG, Rudan D, Rudan I, et al. Comparison of global estimates of prevalence and risk factors for peripheral artery disease in 2000 and 2010: a systematic review and analysis. Lancet (London, England) 2013;382(9901):1329–40.
3. Nehler MR, Duval S, Diao L, et al. Epidemiology of peripheral arterial disease and critical limb ischemia in an insured national population. J Vasc Surg 2014;60(3): 686–95.e2.
4. Hirsch AT, Criqui MH, Treat-Jacobson D, et al. Peripheral arterial disease detection, awareness, and treatment in primary care. JAMA 2001;286(11):1317–24.
5. Sampson UK, Fowkes FG, McDermott MM, et al. Global and regional burden of death and disability from peripheral artery disease: 21 world regions, 1990 to 2010. Global Heart 2014;9(1):145–58.e21.
6. Zwiebel WPJ. Introduction to vascular ultrasonography. Philadelphia, PA: Elsevier Saunders; 2005. p. 253–381.
7. Fowkes FG. The measurement of atherosclerotic peripheral arterial disease in epidemiological surveys. Int J Epidemiol 1988;17(2):248–54.
8. Mohler ER 3rd, Gornik HL, Gerhard-Herman M, et al. ACCF/ACR/AIUM/ASE/ASN/ICAVL/SCAI/SCCT/SIR/SVM/SVS/SVU [corrected] 2012 appropriate use criteria for peripheral vascular ultrasound and physiological testing part I: arterial ultrasound and physiological testing: a report of the American College of Cardiology Foundation appropriate use criteria task force, American College of Radiology, American Institute of Ultrasound in Medicine, American Society of Echocardiography, American Society of Nephrology, Intersocietal Commission for the Accreditation of Vascular Laboratories, Society for Cardiovascular Angiography and Interventions, Society of Cardiovascular Computed Tomography, Society for Interventional Radiology, Society for Vascular Medicine, Society for Vascular Surgery, [corrected] and Society for Vascular Ultrasound. [corrected]. J Am Coll Cardiol 2012;60(3):242–76.
9. Gerhard-Herman MD, Gornik HL, Barrett C, et al. 2016 AHA/ACC Guideline on the Management of Patients with Lower Extremity Peripheral Artery Disease: Executive Summary. Vasc Med 2017;22(3):Np1–43.
10. Choi E, Henkin S. Raynaud's phenomenon and related vasospastic disorders. Vasc Med 2021;26(1):56–70.
11. Nawaz I, Nawaz Y, Nawaz E, et al. Raynaud's Phenomenon: Reviewing the Pathophysiology and Management Strategies. Cureus 2022;14(1):e21681.
12. Das S, Maiti A. Acrocyanosis: an overview. Indian J Dermatol 2013;58(6):417–20.

13. Cleveland. Clinic Non-Invasive Vascular Laboratory Protocols+Procedures. Manual 2019.

14. Scallan J, Huxley VH, Korthuis RJ. Integrated systems physiology: from molecule to function to disease. Capillary fluid exchange: regulation, functions, and Pathology. Morgan & Claypool Life Sciences Copyright © 2010. Philadelphia, PA: Morgan & Claypool Life Sciences; 2010.

15. Gloviczki P, Lawrence PF, Wasan SM, et al. The 2022 Society for Vascular Surgery, American Venous Forum, and American Vein and Lymphatic Society clinical practice guidelines for the management of varicose veins of the lower extremities. Part I. Duplex Scanning and Treatment of Superficial Truncal Reflux: Endorsed by the Society for Vascular Medicine and the International Union of Phlebology. J Vasc Surg Venous Lymphat Disord 2023;11(2):231–61.e6.

16. Dezotti NRA, Dalio MB, Ribeiro MS, et al. The clinical importance of air plethysmography in the assessment of chronic venous disease. J Vasc Bras 2016; 15(4):287–92.

17. Owens DK, Davidson KW, Krist AH, et al. Screening for Abdominal Aortic Aneurysm: US Preventive Services Task Force Recommendation Statement. JAMA 2019;322(22):2211–8.

18. Isselbacher EM, Preventza O, Hamilton Black J Iii, et al. 2022 ACC/AHA Guideline for the Diagnosis and Management of Aortic Disease: A Report of the American Heart Association/American College of Cardiology Joint Committee on Clinical Practice Guidelines. J Am Coll Cardiol 2022;80(24):e223–393.

19. van Walraven C, Wong J, Morant K, et al. Incidence, follow-up, and outcomes of incidental abdominal aortic aneurysms. J Vasc Surg 2010;52(2):282–9, e1-2.

20. Sevil FC, Tort M, Özer Gökaslan Ç, et al. Incidence, follow-up and outcomes of incidental abdominal aortic aneurysms in computed tomography. Interact Cardiovasc Thorac Surg 2022;34(4):645–51.

21. Chaikof EL, Dalman RL, Eskandari MK, et al. The Society for Vascular Surgery practice guidelines on the care of patients with an abdominal aortic aneurysm. J Vasc Surg 2018;67(1):2–77.e2.

22. Krist AH, Davidson KW, Mangione CM, et al. Screening for Asymptomatic Carotid Artery Stenosis: US Preventive Services Task Force Recommendation Statement. JAMA 2021;325(5):476–81.

23. AbuRahma AF, Avgerinos ED, Chang RW, et al. Society for Vascular Surgery clinical practice guidelines for management of extracranial cerebrovascular disease. J Vasc Surg 2022;75(1s):4s–22s.

24. Daghem M, Bing R, Fayad ZA, et al. Noninvasive Imaging to Assess Atherosclerotic Plaque Composition and Disease Activity: Coronary and Carotid Applications. JACC Cardiovascular imaging 2020;13(4):1055–68.

25. Forsyth A, Zamor KC, Cho J, et al. Single-Center Retrospective Review of Carotid Ultrasound Indications and Outcomes. J Vasc Surg 2021;74(3):e191.

26. Naylor AR, Ricco JB, de Borst GJ, et al. Editor's Choice - Management of Atherosclerotic Carotid and Vertebral Artery Disease: 2017 Clinical Practice Guidelines of the European Society for Vascular Surgery (ESVS). Eur J Vasc Endovasc 2018; 55(1):3–81.

27. Strandness DE Jr. Screening for carotid disease and surveillance for carotid restenosis. Semin Vasc Surg 2001;14(3):200–5.

28. Spence JD, Song H, Cheng G. Appropriate management of asymptomatic carotid stenosis. Stroke and vascular neurology 2016;1(2):64–71.

29. Sabeti S, Schlager O, Exner M, et al. Progression of carotid stenosis detected by duplex ultrasonography predicts adverse outcomes in cardiovascular high-risk patients. Stroke 2007;38(11):2887–94.

30. Hackam DG. Optimal Medical Management of Asymptomatic Carotid Stenosis. Stroke 2021;52(6):2191–8.

31. Bogiatzi C, Azarpazhooh MR, Spence JD. Choosing the right therapy for a patient with asymptomatic carotid stenosis. Expet Rev Cardiovasc Ther 2020;18(2): 53–63.

Approach to the Patient with Non-cardiac Leg Swelling

Geno J. Merli, MD, MACP, FSVM, FHM[a],*,
Heather Yenser, MSN, CRNP, AGACNP-BC[b],
Dina Orapallo, MSN, CRNP, AGACNP-BC[b]

KEYWORDS

- Non-cardiac • Leg swelling • History and physical examination • Stemmer's sign
- Medication

KEY POINTS

- Lower extremity swelling either unilateral or bilateral is a frequent reason for outpatient office visit.
- There are 7 important historical question that should be solicited in order to set the stage for the physical examination.
- The differential diagnosis of leg swelling should be divided into unilateral and bilateral leg swelling.
- Lipedema and Lymphedema are 2 separate diagnostic categories since they are not the same disease.

INTRODUCTION

Leg swelling is a common complaint of patients presenting for outpatient primary care clinicians visits. This is a challenging problem not only for the appropriate history and physical but also for the diagnosis and management. In this article, the focus will be on the non-cardiac etiologies for leg swelling.

HISTORY AND PHYSICAL EXAMINATION

There are the initial seven key historical questions that must solicited in order to set the stage for the physical examination. The key points are as follows.

1. When did the swelling begin?

[a] Division Vascular Medicine, Jefferson Vascular Center, Sidney Kimmel Medical College, Thomas Jefferson University Hospitals, Suite 6210, Gibbon Building, 111 South 11th Street, Philadelphia, PA 19107, USA; [b] Division of Vascular Medicine, Department of Surgery, Jefferson Vascular Center, Sidney Kimmel Medical College, Thomas Jefferson University Hospitals, Suite 6210, Gibbon Building, 111 South 11th Street, Philadelphia, PA 19107, USA
* Corresponding author.
E-mail address: Geno.Merli@Jefferson.Edu

Med Clin N Am 107 (2023) 945–961
https://doi.org/10.1016/j.mcna.2023.05.009
0025-7125/23/© 2023 Elsevier Inc. All rights reserved.

2. Where is the swelling located?
3. Does anything make the swelling better?
4. Is the swelling painful or painless
5. Does swelling pit or not pit on finger pressure?
6. Has there been previous lower extremity surgery, trauma (fractures), radiation, joint inflammation, recurrent skin infections, or malignancy
7. What medications is the patient taking?

Begin the history by soliciting approximately when the swelling began. This should be followed by the location either above and/or below the knee as well as the laterality of the swelling. Next ask if anything makes the swelling better. Focus on what the patient has tried to manage the swelling such as elevation, use of support stockings, ace wrapping or use of diuretics. A very important question is whether the swelling is painful or painless. This will assist in differentiation whether inflammation, infection, or thrombosis is the underlying etiology for swelling. Another important point is whether the swelling is pitting or non-pitting. This factor will direct us to the etiology for excess interstitial fluid. It is important to document previous lower extremity surgeries, traumatic injuries such as fractures, radiation, joint inflammation (gout or arthritis), recurrent skin infections or malignancy. Finally review the patient's medication list in order to identify drugs that cause peripheral edema.

The physical examination is centered on the findings of the above seven points. The measurement of leg circumference above and below knee provides discrepancy between the extremities. Next focus on skin discoloration especially redness with increased warmth, or brown hemosiderin pigmentation. The assessment of edema with respect to pitting and non-pitting directs us to causes for increased lower extremity interstitial fluid. Painful pitting edema could indicate swelling secondary to cellulitis, deep vein thrombosis, crystalline, or inflammatory arthropathies. Painless non-pitting edema may be related to lymphatic obstruction either from primary or secondary lymphedema etiologies. In these cases the Stemmer's Sign should be elicited which is pinching the base of the second or third toe[1] (**Fig. 1**) If the skin does not squeeze together this is a positive Stemmer's Sign and indicative of lymphedema. In some cases, there is an enlargement of the extremities from the waist downward with the sparing of the feet. This pattern indicates the diagnosis of lipedema.

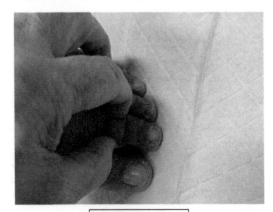

Stemmer's Sign: Pinching the base of the second toe. If the skin does not squeeze together, indicative of Lymphedema.

Fig. 1. Stemmer's sign.

Survey the lower extremities for joint effusions, scars from previous surgeries or traumatic injuries, skin discoloration, varicose veins, healed lower extremity ulcers, and increased skin warmth. Knee swelling with the involvement of the calf may be an indication of a popliteal cyst. Leg swelling involving the entire extremity including the dorsum of the foot is compatible with.

The physical examination of the lower extremity should focus on the size, presence of joint effusions, circulation (venous and arterial), tenderness to palpation, and skin changes.

Patients with congenital venous malformations have hypertrophy of the tissues and bone of the involved limb, giving it an enlarged appearance or a leg length discrepancy[2] Congenital venous malformations are noted as raised, bluish colored vessels isolated to the calf or thigh and do not follow the distribution of the major veins of the extremity. The assessment of the knee joint for excess fluid is an important part of the examination of unilateral leg swelling. Popliteal cysts frequently present with knee effusion in addition to lower extremity swelling. Assessing the patient's popliteal space in the standing position often enhances the appearance of a cyst. The presence of chronic venous insufficiency is manifest by distended veins over the surface of the lower extremity following the distribution of the greater or lesser saphenous veins. Often there are multiple small superficial veins over the foot that are secondary to increased venous pressure caused by retrograde blood flow from incompetent valves.

Patients may present with acute onset of calf pain and swelling and develop a bluish purple discoloration below the medial malleolus. This crescent-shaped skin discoloration is caused by the downward gravitation of blood from either a ruptured popliteal cyst or a tear of the gastrocnemius muscle.[3] In addition, patients with the latter injury are noted to have a sunken area where the muscle is torn on the medial side of the mid-calf on standing.

Patients with a history of chronic lower extremity swelling have skin changes commensurate with the duration of the underlying disease. The skin of patients with lymphedema is dry and scaling. The longer the duration of swelling, the greater thickening of the tissues occurs, with an elephant skin texture and multiple verrucous-like changes. In chronic venous insufficiency, the golden brown hemosiderin deposition is either localized to the distal medial aspect of the ankle or diffuse over the calf.

Unilateral Lower Extremity Swelling

Lymphedema

The diagnosis of lymphedema should be consider in patients with unilateral or bilateral swelling of an extremity secondary to a malformation or obstruction of lymphatic channels (**Fig. 2**). The primary function of the lymphatics is to clear the interstitial space of excess proteinaceous fluid and return it to blood circulation. When this protein-rich fluid is not adequately removed, lymphedema develops. This edema is primarily painless and non-pitting. In these cases, the Stemmer's Sign should be elicited which is pinching the base of the second or third toe[1] (see **Fig. 1**). If the skin does not squeeze together this is a positive Stemmer's Sign and indicative of lymphedema.[1] Lymphedema can be classified into 2 categories primary and secondary types (**Tables 1** and **2**).

Primary lymphedema is considered a clinical manifestation of a lymphatic malformation developed during the later stage of lymphangiogensis. The primary lymphedemas included congenital, praecox, and tarda.[4] The first category is Nonne-Milroy disease, congenital hereditary lymphedema, diagnosed in patients presenting at birth or within the first 2 years of life, has an autosomal-dominant inheritance, and can cause bilateral lower extremity lymphedema and intestinal lymphangiectasia and

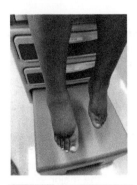 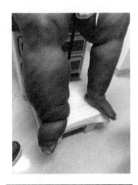 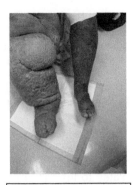

Early Stage of Lymphedema	Later Stage of Lymphedema	End Stage of Lymphedema
Painless, Non-Pitting edema	Painless, Non-Pitting edema	Painless, Non-Pitting edema
		Severe hypertrophy of skin

Fig. 2. Lymphedema.

cholestasis.[5] It is associated with an inactivation mutation of the vascular endothelial growth factor receptor 3 tyrosine kinase signaling pathway found in lymphatic vessels.[6,7] The second category is Meige disease, familial lymphedema praecox, presents during puberty. Other clinical manifestations are cerebrovascular malformations, vertebral defects, hearing problems, and distichiasis.[8] It is associated with sequence variations in the human forkhead box C2 (FOXC2) gene, a transcription factor in adipocyte metabolism, and has an autosomal-dominant inheritance.[9] The third category is a late-onset type, lymphedema tarda, usually presents after age.[10]

Secondary lymphedema is more prevalent and develops when intact lymphatics become obstructed or obliterated such as the following: infections, inflammatory, surgical, radiation, or traumatic injury. Filarial infection in countries with developing economies remains the most prevalent cause of secondary lymphedema.[11] In countries with affluent economies, lymphatic resection and irradiation for staging or regional

Table 1 Primary lymphedema	
Types Primary Lymphedema	**Key Points**
Congenital Hereditary Lymphedema (Nonne-Milroy Disease)	Presents at birth or within the first 2 years of life, has an autosomal-dominant inheritance, and can cause bilateral lower extremity lymphedema and intestinal lymphangiectasia and cholestasis. It is associated with an inactivation mutation of the vascular endothelial growth factor receptor 3 tyrosine kinase signaling pathway found in lymphatic vessels.
Familial Lymphedema Praecox (Meige disease)	Presents during puberty. Other clinical manifestations are cerebrovascular malformations, vertebral defects, hearing problems, and distichiasis. It is associated with sequence variations in the human forkhead box C2 (FOXC2) gene, a transcription factor in adipocyte metabolism, and has an autosomal-dominant inheritance.
Lymphedema Tarda, (Late-Onset Type)	Usually present after the age of 35 years

Table 2
Secondary lymphedema

Secondary Lymphedema	Etiologies
Obstructive	Tumor
	Trauma (crush injury)
Obliterative	Surgery
	Tumor
	Radiation
	Sarcoidosis
Inflammatory	Parasitic Infection
	Bacterial Infection

cancer control is the most common cause.[12] More recently the obesity pandemic has produced a rapidly expanding subgroup of patients with lymphedema in the setting of obesity and lack other etiologies for lymphatic compromise.[13,14] Secondary lymphedema is predominantly unilateral, non-pitting, painless or painful and regresses slowly with elevation. The patient's history is probably the most important factor in differentiating the etiology for secondary lymphedemas.

The workup of these patients requires a history and physical examination, supplemented by laboratory tests as indicated. Computed tomography or MR imaging of the abdomen and pelvis may supplement the physical examination in differentiating primary versus secondary lymphedema. Decongestive therapy is the mainstay of lymphedema management no matter the etiology. It consists of movement exercises, manual lymphatic drainage, and compression therapy (bandaging, garments, intermittent of sequential pneumatic compression). The goal of lymphedema therapy is to improve the physical characteristics of the limb and the quality of life.

ACUTE DEEP VEIN THROMBOSIS

Venous thrombosis, comprising deep vein thrombosis (DVT) and pulmonary embolism (PE), occurs with an incidence of approximately 1 per 1000 annually in adult populations (**Fig. 3**).[15] Rates are slightly higher in men than women. About two-thirds of episodes manifest as DVT and one-third as PE with or without DVT.[16] Deep vein thrombosis is an important etiology to consider in a patient presenting with unilateral leg swelling. This is an important diagnosis because of the risk thromboembolic event which can occur because of the thromboembolic risk. In the patient presenting to the outpatient office with unilateral leg swelling, consideration of deep vein thrombosis in the differential diagnosis is significant because of the risk of thromboembolic events. The solicitation of key points in the history is of major importance in considering deep vein thrombosis as a cause of unilateral leg swelling. First, an inciting event should always be sought, such as a recent surgery, prolonged immobilization, or trauma. Further questioning should probe for previous episodes of thrombosis and their inciting events, medications, personal history of malignancy, a family history of thrombosis, and concomitant medical illnesses. The most common presentation of deep vein thrombosis is the acute onset of unilateral leg swelling and pain. The pain may be exacerbated by weight bearing or ambulation. Patients often describe their extremity as either tight, knot-like, or vice-like pain or aching pain deep in the extremity. The edema is localized in the foot and ankle but progresses upward depending on the extent of the underlying thrombosis. This edema is pitting in character but develops a peau de orange

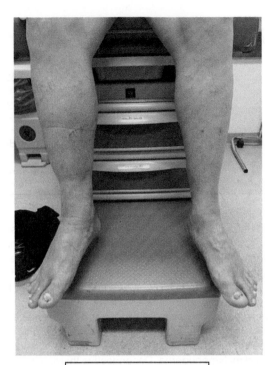

Right Lower extremity enlarged

Fig. 3. Acute deep vein thrombosis.

consistency when the venous return is severely impaired. The extremity has an increased warmth and may often be red or discolored. The measurement of the extremity circumference from a designated point above and below the knee documents the degree of swelling. This will be used to assess the degree of symptomatic improvement. Although many of these signs are poorly sensitive and specific, they may help raise a clinical suspicion in the future of deep vein thrombosis warranting further diagnostic testing. At present, noninvasive Doppler ultrasonography is the accepted method for detecting lower extremity deep vein thrombosis. The cardinal sign is the identification of an area of non-compressibility along the course of the interrogated vessels.[17]

POSTTHROMBOTIC SYNDROME

Post Thrombotic Syndrome (PTS) develops in 20% to 50% of patients within 2 years of DVT diagnosis and is severe in 5% to 10% of cases (**Fig. 4**).[18]

The clinical manifestations of PTS comprise a constellation of symptoms and signs that vary between patients[18] Typical PTS symptoms include leg pain; sensations of leg heaviness, pulling, or fatigue; and limb swelling. These symptoms can be manifested in different combinations such as persistent or intermittent which can be aggravated by standing or walking but improve with rest and leg elevation. Typical signs may include single leg edema, redness, dusky cyanosis when the leg is in a dependent position, medial malleolar reticular veins, new varicose veins, skin thickening, and hyperpigmentation known as lipodermatosclerosis, and in severe cases, leg ulcers.[18] These ulcers are characteristically painful and slow healing. The intensity of symptoms and

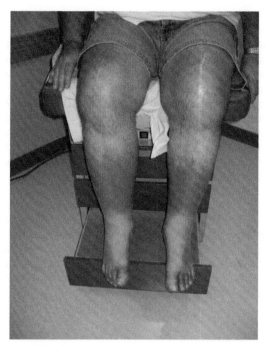

Fig. 4. Postthrombotic syndrome.

signs increase with weight bearing and can vary from minimal to severe with chronic pain, swelling, and leg ulceration.

The risk of PTS is 2 to threefold higher after proximal than distal DVT. Other risk factors for PTS include the following: Previous ipsilateral DVT, Preexisting primary venous insufficiency (up to twofold risk), elevated body mass index > 30 (doubles the risk), older age (30% to 3 fold).[19,20] The following factors appear to have little or no effect on the risk of developing PTS: sex, whether DVT was provoked vs unprovoked and biological thrombophilia.

PTS is believed to develop following DVT secondary to venous hypertension. Venous hypertension reduces calf muscle perfusion which increases tissue permeability and promotes the clinical manifestations of PTS. Two pathologic mechanisms contribute to venous hypertension: persistent acute followed by residual venous obstruction and valvular reflux secondary to damaged vein valves[21] Anticoagulant treatment of DVT prevents clot propagation and pulmonary embolization but does not lyse the clot leaving residual venous scarring. Inflammation may play a role in promoting the development of PTS by delaying thrombus resolution and by inducing vein wall fibrosis, which promotes valvular reflux.[22,23]

Because recurrent DVT is a strong risk factor for PTS, optimal intensity and duration of anticoagulation is an important clinical goal. Unfortunately, there is insufficient data to make specific recommendations regarding the choice of anticoagulant to treat DVT, namely a vitamin K antagonist versus a direct oral anticoagulant versus LMWH monotherapy, on the outcome of developing PTS.

The data on the use of gradient elastic stockings in patients with DVT to prevent PTS has been conflicting. In the past, evidence-based consensus guidelines recommended the use of ECS for at least 2 years after DVT. A recent meta-analysis that incorporated data from the SOX Trial reported a pooled hazard ratio for PTS with ECS of

0.69 (95% confidence interval [CI], 0.47-1.02). However, the authors caution that there is very low confidence in this pooled estimate because of heterogeneity and inclusion of unblinded studies at high risk of bias, and that the recent, highest-quality evidence available suggests no effect of ECS on PTS.[24] Based on these new data, the latest guideline statements do not advocate the routine use of ECS to prevent PTS.[18,25] Although ECS are unlikely to cause harm, they can be difficult to apply, uncomfortable, expensive, and require replacement every few months. Since lower extremity swelling makes wearing 20-30 mm Hg knee high gradient elastic stockings placing and removing them difficult and the above data on the efficacy, I opt to use tubigrip knee high to control swelling. This is material provided 15 mm Hg pressure and can be doubled to provide 30 mm Hg as swelling decreases. We eventually convert the patient to knee high 20-30 mm Hg gradient elastic stockings as long as the patient derives symptomatic benefit or is able to tolerate them.

A recent systematic review and meta-analysis evaluated the effectiveness of "venoactive" drugs for PTS.[26] The drugs evaluated were rutosides, defibrotide and hidrosmin.

This meta-analysis did not support the use of vasoactive agents in PTS because of the inconsistency and duration of the therapies. We do not use these agents in the management of PTS. Severe PTS develops in 5% to 10% of patients which may progress to ulceration. This group of patient should be referred to wound care center for multicomponent compression bandaging and debridement as needed.[27]

RUPTURED POPLITEAL CYST

Ruptured Popliteal cyst (Baker's cyst) is another cause to be considered in the differential diagnosis of unilateral leg swelling. The incidence of this anatomic abnormality of the knee has been reported by magnetic resonance (MR) imaging to be approximately 5%.[28] These cysts are more commonly observed in patients with inflammatory joint disease, such as rheumatoid arthritis.[29] Non-inflammatory diseases constitute the second major group with entities such as degenerative joint disease, tears of the posterior horn of the medial meniscus, and knee trauma[28,29] The most frequent clinical manifestation of popliteal cysts are calf pain, swelling, and knee effusion. These symptoms and signs result because popliteal cysts are connected to the gastrocnemius-semimembranous bursa in the calf. Evidence has shown a one-way valve effect in which fluid can go from the knee to the popliteal synovial bursa but not in the reverse direction.[30] These cysts are usually seen along the medial side of the popliteal fossa, distal to the transverse skin crease. Occasionally a crescent sign has been observed along the base of the medial malleolus. These signs and symptoms occur acutely with a large number of cysts either dissecting into the calf or rupturing with blood traversing downward to the ankle via the fascial planes. Doppler ultrasound and MR imaging have demonstrated a nearly equal sensitivity and specificity and are noninvasive. Doppler ultrasound is the test that may be useful initially because this would rule out the diagnosis of thrombosis and allow the interrogation of the popliteal space. If knee derangement is the major concern, MR imaging can be performed.

Although there is a large variety of treatment methods described, the literature remains clear that the mainstay of initial treatment for popliteal cysts is conservative management with.

Corticosteroid Injection if Persistently Symptomatic

A recent systematic review of popliteal cyst management recommended the use of ultrasound evaluation to identify simple cysts compared with complex cysts, with intracystic aspiration and corticosteroid injection and possible cyst fenestration for complex cysts as the best management.[31] Operative management should be reserved for persistently symptomatic cysts and treatment must include addressing the primary intra articular pathology in addition to the cyst itself.[31] The current literature suggests that the arthroscopic enlargement of the cyst opening with the debridement of the cyst wall is an effective technique with the least recurrences.[32]

RUPTURE OF THE MEDIAL HEAD OF THE GASTROCNEMIUS MUSCLE

An acute tear of the medial head of the gastrocnemius muscle closely mimics acute thrombosis of the deep vein system of the calf. Important points in the history and physical examination may help make this differentiation easier for the clinician. Frequently, this injury occurs in middle-aged patients during the process of sudden dorsiflexion of the ankle while extending the knee joint or dorsiflexion while the foot is planted on the ground.[33,34] Pain in the medial aspect of the mid-calf area is acute in onset. This pain may be described by some patients as a sensation of tearing or popping in the calf. Over a 24- to 48-hour period, swelling develops in the calf and ankle areas. Occasionally a bluish discoloration of the lower medial aspect of the ankle may occur owing to the downward movement of blood along the fascial planes from the initial tear. Performing Homan's sign, palpating the gastrocnemius muscle for cords, standing, and walking all produce pain and tenderness in the central portion of the calf. Sometimes a small sunken area may be visible or palpable on the medial side of the mid-calf, where there is pain and tenderness.[35,36] The diagnosis of a tear of the medial head of the gastrocnemius muscle is primarily made by the history and physical examination. If testing is indicated, venous duplex scanning is recommended to rule out deep vein thrombosis or popliteal cyst. MR imaging and computed tomography have been used to evaluate this process but are costly for routine use.

Bilateral Lower Extremity Swelling

Medication-related edema
Calcium channel blockers. Hypertension is the most common chronic condition in the United States, occurring in nearly 50% of all adults **(Fig. 5)**.[37] Calcium channel blockers (CCBs) are a major drug class of vasodilator medications for treating hypertension and linked to drug-related lower extremity swelling. A predominant side effect of CCBs is the formation of peripheral edema.[38] The mechanism for this dose-dependent edema formation is related to the ability of CCBs to selectively dilate arterioles in the absence of venous dilation, ultimately leading to increased capillary

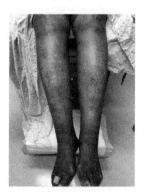

Medication Induced Edema

Bilateral lower extremity swelling two weeks after initiating amlodipine for hypertension management

Bilateral Post Thrombotic Syndrome

Patient 5 years post bilateral Total Knee Arthroplasty. Swelling and pigmentation present bilaterally

Fig. 5. Medication induces extremity swelling.

pressure and extravasation of interstitial fluid.[39,40] A predominant side effect of CCBs is the formation of peripheral edema.[38]

Dihydropyridine calcium channel blockers (DH CCBs) are prescribed to approximately 1 in 5 adults with hypertension in the United States and are considered a first-line option given their cardiovascular benefits.[41,42] Dihydropyridine calcium channel blockers are also generally considered safe because they do not require routine electrolyte or kidney function monitoring, nor do they cause diuresis.[43,44] A disadvantage to their use is the risk of lower-extremity edema, a dose-dependent and duration-dependent adverse event with an estimated incidence of 12%.[38,44,45] The preferred treatment for DH CCB–induced edema includes DH CCB dose reduction or discontinuation, which typically reduces or completely resolves the edema.[44,45]

Thiazodilinediones

Thiazodilinediones are used for the treatment of type II diabetes, but one of their side effects is lower extremity edema that occurs in a dose-dependent manner.[46] In clinical trials the incidence of edema was 3.0 to 7.5% in patients taking TZDs as a solo medication versus placebo or other antidiabetic agents. TZD in combination with insulin has been shown to increase the incidence of peripheral edema to 15.3% with pioglitazone and 14.7% in the rosiglitazone group.[47] The mechanisms responsible for this drug-related edema are unclear, but a limited number of studies indicate that TZDs may directly affect lymphatic function. In all the above studies, the peripheral edema failed to respond to diuretics while on the thiazolidinediones. It was the discontinuation of these agents that impacted the peripheral edema. It was postulated that the thiazolidinediones may have some effect on the delivery of diuretics to the lumen of the nephron or may induce tubular alterations that impair the ability of the nephrons to respond to diuretics.

Peripheral edema is a class effect of the thiazolidinediones and is multifactorial in origin. This edema is dose related and is increased when used in combination with insulin therapy. It is recommended to initiate these agents at low dose and follow the patients closely of peripheral edema. Diuretics do not work for this type of edema. The discontinuation of the thiazolidinediones is recommended as the management.

NON-STEROIDAL ANTI-INFLAMMATORY DRUGS

Non-Steroidal Anti-Inflammatory Drugs (NSAID) are commonly used agents for the treatment of joint aches and pains. Peripheral edema has been reported in 2-5% of patients taking these agents especially the elderly or those with volume depletion.[48] The primary mechanism NSAIDs is the inhibition of the cyclooxygenase-dependent generation of prostaglandins which disrupts renal homeostasis. COX-1 and COX-2 synthesize PGE2 and PGI2, which are both involved in NSAID-associated peripheral edema.[49,50] NSAID-induced PGE2 lowering decreases both natriuresis in the thick ascending loop of Henle and aquaresis through the facilitation of arginine vasopressin activity in the collecting duct.[49-51] NSAIDs inhibit PGI2-related afferent arteriole vasodilatation, reducing the glomerular filtration rate and thus promoting proximal tubular reabsorption.[51] Nonselective and COX-2 selective NSAIDs have similar incidences of peripheral edema, supporting the finding that fluid retention is mostly COX-2 mediated.[48-51] The edema from NSAID is mild and usually manifests in the first week of use and is reversible on the discontinuation of the agent.

LIPEDEMA

Lipedema was first reported by Drs Allen and Hines in the United States (**Fig. 6**).[52] It is a chronic, progressive disorder that predominantly affects women versus men.

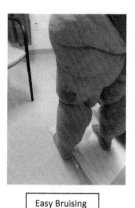

Easy Bruising

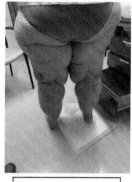

Sparing of Feet

Ankle pronation

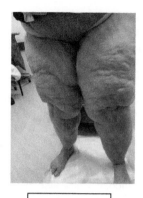

Dimpling of Skin

Fig. 6. Lipedema.

Lipedema develops a symmetrical painless enlargement of subcutaneous adipose tissue of the extremities is characteristic for lipohypertrophy.[53] A trigger for the development of lipedema tissue may be an increase in fluid and connective tissue remodeling that occurs alongside body changes during puberty, childbirth, menopause, stress associated with lifestyle change, or by altering tissue structure after surgery or trauma.[54]

Lipedema is characterized by the abnormal distribution of adipose tissue which results in a pronounced disproportion between extremities and trunk. There are three stages of Lipedema listed in **Table 3**. Other findings include the following: edema aggravated by orthostasis, easy bruising following minor trauma, increased tenderness to pressure, and pain syndromes. A hallmark of lipedema tissue is inflammation resulting in tissue fibrosis and pain, and in some cases, the tissue may become numb. The prevalence of lipedema has been estimated as high as 10% in adult Caucasian women.[55]

The major finding on physical examination is the disproportionate distribution of adipose tissue. This could involve the lower extremities with buttocks and thighs, thighs only, or the entire extremities. The skin has a velvet-like consistency with dimpling. The feet and hands are spare. The Stemmer's sign is negative. The ankles are pronated. There is a cut off sign at the ankles bilaterally. Lipedema is often confused with obesity, as the BMI increases due to the swollen extremities. However, the adipose tissue in lipedema is resistant to exercise or diet. As in lipedema, lipohypertrophy is

Table 3 Lipedema	
Stages **Lipedema**	**Characteristics**
Stage 1	Smooth skin, soft homogenous increase in subcutaneous tissue, cool skin in certain areas because of functional vascular imbalance
Stage 2	Irregular skin surface, nodular changes of the subcutaneous tissue
Stage 3	Tender subcutaneous nodules, pronounced increase in circumference with loose skin/tissue, bulging protrusion of fat mainly at inner thighs and knees

seen in females only. It has a negative esthetic impact but misses the sufferings that are so characteristic of lipedema. The most common comorbidity in lipohypertrophy patients in obesity with 80% of affected patient.[53]

CHRONIC VENOUS INSUFFICIENCY

Chronic venous insufficiency (CVI) describes a condition that affects the venous system of the lower extremities, with the *sine qua non* being persistent ambulatory venous hypertension causing various pathologies, including pain, edema, skin changes, and ulcerations (**Fig. 7**).[56] CVI often indicates the more advanced forms of venous disorders, including manifestations such as hyperpigmentation, venous eczema, lipodermatosclerosis, atrophie blanche, and healed or active ulcers. However, because varicose veins also have incompetent valves and increased venous pressure, we use the term "CVI" to represent the full spectrum of manifestations of chronic venous disease.[57]

Risk factors found to be associated with CVI include age, sex, a family history of varicose veins, obesity, pregnancy, phlebitis, and previous leg injury[58,59] There are also environmental or behavioral factors associated with CVI, such as prolonged standing and perhaps a sitting posture at work.[60,61]

The more serious consequences of CVI it the development of venous ulcers which have an estimated prevalence of 0.3%.[61] It has been estimated that approximately 2.5 million people experience CVI in the United States, and of those approximately 20% develop venous ulcers.[62] The overall prognosis of venous ulcers is poor, because delayed healing and recurrent ulceration are very common[63] Disability related to venous ulcers leads to loss of productive work hours, estimated at 2 million workdays per year, and may cause early retirement, found in >12% of workers with venous

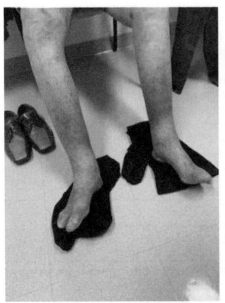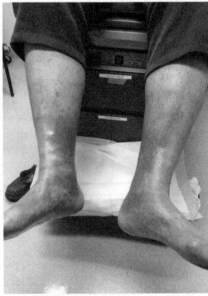

Bilateral Chronic Venous Insufficiency

Fig. 7. Chronic venous insufficiency.

ulcers[64] The financial burden of venous ulcer disease on the healthcare system is readily apparent, with an estimated $1 billion spent annually on the treatment of chronic wounds in the United States[65,66] The Clinical Practice Guidelines (CPG) of the Society for Vascular Surgery and American Venous Forum of 2011 provided the best evidence-based practice for clinicians.[67]

The physical examination is important in establishing the diagnosis of CVI. The skin is examined for prominent, dilated superficial venous abnormalities, such as telangiectasis, reticular veins, or varicose veins. The distribution of these varicose veins may follow the course of the affected superficial vein, such as the GSV and lesser saphenous vein. This evaluation should include positioning in the upright posture to allow for the maximal distention of the veins. Additional skin findings may be seen, such as hyperpigmentation, stasis dermatitis, atrophie blanche, or lipodermatosclerosis. The edema seen in CVI is dependent and usually pitting. An early finding of venous congestion includes calf fullness or increased limb girth for which extremity circumference should be measured. The presence of active or healed ulcers near the medial aspect of the ankle with GSV reflux or lateral aspects of the ankle with lesser saphenous vein reflux, may be seen with more advanced disease.[68]

The initial management of CVI involves conservative measures to reduce symptoms and prevent the development of secondary complications and progression of disease. The use of compressive stockings is the mainstay of conservative management and is further described later in discussion. If conservative measures fail, referral to a vascular medicine or vascular surgeon is recommended.

CLINICS CARE POINTS

- In the United States secondary lymphedema is the most common eitiology of leg swelling.
- Acute Deep Vein Thrombosis presents as painful unilateral leg swelling associated secondary risk factors.
- Post Thrombotic Syndrome develops in 20% to 50% of patients within 2 years of the DVT diagnosis.
- Medications are one of the most common causes of bilateral leg swelling with calcium channel blockers being high on the list.
- Lipedema is a disproportionate distribution of adipose tissue is the major finding in this disorder.
- The history and physical examination are key to differentiating Lymphedema and Lipedma.
- Valvular dysfunction is the etiology for chronic venous insufficiency.

DISCLOSURE

The authors have nothing to disclose.

REFERENCES

1. Gross JA, Greene AK. Sensitivity and specificity of the Stemmer Sign for lymphedema: a clinical Lymphoscintigraphic study. Plast Reconstr Surg Glob Open 2019;7(6):e2295.
2. John P. Kippel Trenaunay Syndrome Tech Vasc Interv Radiol 2019;22(4):100634.

3. Good AE, Pozderac RV. Ecchymosis of the lower leg. A sign of haemarthrosis with synovial rupture. Arthritis Rheum 1977;20:1009–13.

4. Manrique OJ, Bustos SS, Ciudad P, et al. Overview of lymphedema for physicians and other clinicians: a review of fundamental concepts. Mayo Clin Proc 2022; 97(10):1920–35.

5. Smeltzer DM, Stickler GB, Schirger A. Primary lymphedema in children and adolescents: a follow-up study and review. Pediatrics 1985;76(2):206–18.

6. Irrthum A, Karkkainen MJ, Devriendt K, et al. Congenital hereditary lymphedema caused by a mutation that inactivates VEGFR3 tyrosine kinase. Am J Hum Genet 2000;67(2):295–301.

7. Karkkainen MJ, Ferrell RE, Lawrence EC, et al. Missense mutations interfere with VEGFR-3 signalling in primary lymphoedema. Nat Genet 2000;25(2): 153–9.

8. Wheeler ES, Chan V, Wassman R, et al. Familial lymphedema praecox: meige's disease. Plast Reconstr Surg 1981;67(3):362–4.

9. Yildirim-Toruner C, Subramanian K, El Manjra L, et al. A novel frameshift mutation of FOXC2 gene in a family with hereditary lymphedemadistichiasis syndrome associated with renal disease and diabetes mellitus. Am J Med Genet 2004; 131(3):281–6.

10. Connell F, Brice G, Jeffery S, et al. A new classification system for primary lymphatic dysplasias based on phenotype. Clin Genet 2010;77(5):438–52.

11. Ramaiah KD, Ottesen EA. Progress and impact of 13 years of the global programme to eliminate lymphatic filariasis on reducing the burden of filarial disease. PLoS Neglected Trop Dis 2014;8(11).

12. Laredo J, Lee BB. Lymphedema. In: Mowatt-Larssen E, Desai SS, Dua A, et al, editors. Phlebology, vein surgery and ultrasonography: diagnosis and management of venous disease. Cham, Switzerland: Springer International Publishing; 2014. p. 327–39.

13. Cederberg A, Grønning LM, Ahrén B, et al. FOXC2 is a winged helix gene that counteracts obesity, hypertriglyceridemia, and diet-induced insulin resistance. Cell 2001;106(5):563–73.

14. Mehrara BJ, Greene AK. Lymphedema and obesity: is there a link? Plast Reconstr Surg 2014;134(1):154e–60e.

15. Cushman M. Epidemiology and risk factors for venous thrombosis. Semin Hematol 2007;44(2):62–9.

16. Cushman M, Tsai AW, White RH, et al. Deep vein thrombosis and pulmonary embolism in two cohorts: the Longitudinal Investigation of Thromboembolism Etiology. Am J Med 2004;117:19–25.

17. Needleman L, Cronan J, Lilly M, et al. Ultrasound for lower extremity deep venous thrombosis: multidisciplinary recommendations from the society of radiologists in ultrasound consensus conference. Circulation 2018;137(14): 1505–15, 3.

18. Kahn SR, Comerota AJ, Cushman M, et al. American heart association council on peripheral vascular disease, council on clinical cardiology and council on cardiovascular and stroke nursing. the postthrombotic syndrome: evidence-based prevention, diagnosis, and treatment strategies: a scientific statement from the American heart association. Circulation 2014;130(18): 1636–61.

19. Rabinovich A, Kahn SR. How to predict and diagnose postthrombotic syndrome. Pol Arch Med Wewn 2014;124(7–8):410–6.

20. Galanaud J-P, Monreal M, Kahn SR. Predictors of the post-thrombotic syndrome and their effect on the therapeutic management of deep vein thrombosis. J Vasc Surg Venous Lymphat Disord 2016;4(4):531–4.

21. Vedantham S. Valvular dysfunction and venous obstruction in the postthrombotic syndrome. Thromb Res 2009;123(Suppl 4):S62–5.

22. Deatrick KB, Elfline M, Baker N, et al. Postthrombotic vein wallremodeling: preliminary observations. J Vasc Surg 2011;53(1):139–46.

23. Rabinovich A, Cohen JM, Cushman M, et al. Inflammation markers and their trajectories after deep vein thrombosis in relation to risk of postthrombotic syndrome. J Thromb Haemostasis 2015;13(3):398–408.

24. Berntsen CF, Kristiansen A, Akl EA, et al. Compression stockings for preventing the postthrombotic syndrome in patients with deep vein thrombosis. Am J Med 2016;129(4):447.e1–20.

25. Kearon C, Akl EA, Ornelas J, et al. Antithrombotic therapy for VTE disease: CHEST Guideline and Expert Panel Report. Chest 2016;149(2):315–52.

26. Cohen JM, Akl EA, Kahn SR. Pharmacologic and compression therapies for postthrombotic syndrome: a systematic review of randomized controlled trials. Chest 2012;141(2):308–20.

27. O'Donnell TF Jr, Passman MA, Marston WA, et al, Society for Vascular Surgery; American Venous Forum. Management of venous leg ulcers: clinical practice guidelines of the Society for Vascular Surgery® and the American Venous Forum. J Vasc Surg 2014;60(2 Suppl):3S–59S.

28. Hayashi D, Roemer FW, Dhina Z, et al. Longitudinal assessment of cyst-like lesions of the knee and their relation to radiographic osteoarthritis and MRI-detected effusion and synovitis in patients with knee pain. Arthritis Res Ther 2010;12(5):R172.

29. Liao ST, Chiou CS, Chang CC. Pathology associated to the Baker's cysts: a musculoskeletal ultrasound study. Clin Rheumatol 2010;29:1043–7.

30. Herman AM, Marzo JM. Popliteal cysts: a current review. Orthopedics 2014; 37(8):e678–84.

31. Van Nest DS, Tjoumakaris FP, Smith BJ, et al. Popliteal cysts: a systematic review of nonoperative and operative treatment. JBJS REVIEWS 2020;8(3):e0139.

32. Zhou X, Li B, Wang J, et al. Jo Surgical treatment of popliteal cyst: a systematic review and meta-analysis. J Orthop Surg Res 2016;11:22.

33. Froimson AI. Tennis leg. JAMA 1969;209:415–6.

34. Gilbert TJ, Bullis BR, Griffiths HJ. Tennis calf or tennis leg. Orthopedics 1996; 19:179.

35. Miller WA. Rupture of the musculotendinous juncture of the medial head of the gastrocnemius muscle. Am J Sports Med 1977;5:191–3.

36. Delgado GJ, Chung CB, Lektrakul N, et al. Tennis leg: clinical US study of 141 patients and anatomic investigation of four cadavers with MR imaging and US. Radiology 2002;224:112–9.

37. Benjamin EJ, Muntner P, Alonso A, et al. American Heart Association Council on Epidemiology and Prevention Statistics Committee and Stroke Statistics Subcommittee. Heart disease and stroke statistics 2019 update: a report from the American Heart Association. Circulation 2019;139(10):e56–528.

38. Makani H, Bangalore S, Romero J, et al. Peripheral edema associated with calcium channel blockers: incidence and withdrawal rate – a meta-analysis of randomized trials. J Hypertens 2011;29:1270–80.

39. Zanchetti A, Omboni S, La Commare P, et al. Efficacy, tolerability, and impact on quality of life of long-term treatment with manidipine or amlodipine in patients with essential hypertension. J Cardiovasc Pharmacol 2001;38:642–50.

40. Whelton PK, Carey RM, Aronow WS, et al. 2017 ACC/AHA/AAPA/ABC/ACPM/AGS/APhA/ASH/ASPC/NMA/PCNA guideline for the prevention, detection, evaluation, and management of high blood pressure in adults: a report of the American College of Cardiology/American Heart Association Task Force on Clinical Practice Guidelines. Hypertension 2018;71(6):e13–115.

41. Gu Q, Burt VL, Dillon CF, et al. Trends in antihypertensive medication use and blood pressure control among United States adults with hypertension: the National Health And Nutrition Examination Survey, 2001 to 2010. Circulation 2012; 126(17):2105–14.

42. Neal B, MacMahon S, Chapman N. Blood Pressure Lowering Treatment Trialists' Collaboration. Effects of ACE inhibitors, calcium antagonists, and other blood-pressure-lowering drugs: results of prospectively designed overviews of randomised trials: Blood Pressure Lowering Treatment Trialists' Collaboration. Lancet 2000;356(9246):1955–64.

43. Messerli FH. Vasodilatory edema: a common side effect of antihypertensive therapy. Am J Hypertens 2001;14(9, pt 1):978–9.

44. Messerli FH. Vasodilatory edema: a common side effect of antihypertensive therapy. Curr Cardiol Rep 2002;4(6):479–82.

45. Vouri S, Jiang X, Manini T, et al. Magnitude of and characteristics associated with the treatment of calcium channel blocker-induced lower extremity edema with loop diuretics. JAMA Netw Open 2019;2(12):e 1918425.

46. Mudaliar S, Chang AR, Henry RR. Thiazolidinediones, peripheral edema, and type 2 diabetes: incidence, pathophysiology, and clinical implications. Endocr Pract 2003;9(5):406–16.

47. Scheen AJ. Combined thiazolidinedione-insulin therapy: should we be concerned about safety? Drug Saf 2004;27:841–56.

48. Walker C, Biasucci LM. Cardiovascular safety of non-steroidal anti-inflammatory drugs revisited. Postgrad Med 2018;130(1):55–71.

49. Whelton A. Renal and related cardiovascular effects of conventional and COX-2-specific NSAIDs and non-NSAID analgesics. Am J Ther 2000;7(2):63–74.

50. Cabassi A, Tedeschi S, Perlini S, et al. Non-steroidal anti-inflammatory drug effects on renal and cardiovascular function: from physiology to clinical practice. Eur J Prev Cardiol 2020;27(8):850–67.

51. Frishman WH. Effects of nonsteroidal anti-inflammatory drug therapy on blood pressure and peripheral edema. Am J Cardiol 2002;89(6A):18D–25D.

52. Allen EV, Hines EA Jr. Lipedema of the legs: a syndrome characterized by fat legs and orthostatic edema. Proc Staff Meet Mayo Clin 1940;15:184.

53. Herbst K, Kahn L, Iker E, et al. Standard of care for lipedema in the United States. Phlebology 2021;36(10):779–96.

54. Buck DW 2nd, Herbst KL. Lipedema: a relatively common disease with extremely common misconceptions. Plast Reconstr Surg Glob Open 2016;4:e1043.

55. Wollina U. Lipedema: an update. Dermatol Ther 2019;32:e 12805.

56. Eberhardt RT, Rafetto JD. Chronic venous insufficiency. Circulation 2014;130: 333–46.

57. McLafferty RB, Passman MA, Caprini JA, et al. Increasing awareness about venous disease: the American Venous Forum expands the National Venous Screening Program. J Vasc Surg 2008;48:394–9.

58. Scott TE, LaMorte WW, Gorin DR, et al. Risk factors for chronic venous insufficiency: a dual case-control study. J Vasc Surg 1995;22:622–8.
59. Jawien A. The influence of environmental factors in chronic venous insufficiency. Angiology 2003;54:S19–31.
60. Lacroix P, Aboyans V, Preux PM, et al. Epidemiology of venous insufficiency in an occupational population. Int Angiol 2003;22:172–6.
61. Fowkes FG, Evans CJ, Lee AJ. Prevalence and risk factors for chronic venous insufficiency. Angiology 2001;52:S5–15.
62. Rhodes JM, Gloviczki P, Canton LG, et al. Factors affecting clinical outcome following endoscopic perforator vein ablation. Am J Surg 1998;176:162–7.
63. Callam MJ, Harper DR, Dale JJ, et al. Chronic ulcer of the leg: clinical history. BMJ 1987;294:1389–91.
64. Da Silva A, Navarro MF, Batalheiro J. The importance of chronic venous insufficiency: various preliminary data on its medico-social consequences. Phlebologie 1992;45:439–43.
65. Laing W. Chronic venous disease of the leg. London, United Kingdom: Office of Health Economics; 1992:1–44.Pierce GF, Mustoe TA. Pharmacologic enhancement of wound healing. Annu Rev Med 1995;46:467–81.
66. Pierce GF, Mustoe TA. Pharmacologic enhancement of wound healing. Annu Rev Med 1995;46:467–81.
67. Gloviczki P, Comerota AJ, Dalsing MC, et al. Society for Vascular Surgery; American Venous Forum. The care of patients with varicose veins and associated chronic venous diseases: clinical practice guidelines of the Society for Vascular Surgery and the American Venous Forum. J Vasc Surg 2011;53(5 suppl):2S–48S.
68. Labropoulos N, Leon M, Nicolaides AN, et al. Superficial venous insufficiency: correlation of anatomic extent of reflux with clinical symptoms and signs. J Vasc Surg 1994;20:953–8.

Moving?

Make sure your subscription moves with you!

To notify us of your new address, find your **Clinics Account Number** (located on your mailing label above your name), and contact customer service at:

Email: journalscustomerservice-usa@elsevier.com

800-654-2452 (subscribers in the U.S. & Canada)
314-447-8871 (subscribers outside of the U.S. & Canada)

Fax number: 314-447-8029

Elsevier Health Sciences Division
Subscription Customer Service
3251 Riverport Lane
Maryland Heights, MO 63043

*To ensure uninterrupted delivery of your subscription, please notify us at least 4 weeks in advance of move.

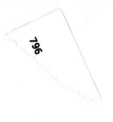

Printed and bound by CPI Group (UK) Ltd, Croydon, CR0 4YY

03/10/2024

01040473-0017